DE HISTORIA
UROLOGIAE EUROPAEAE

DE HISTORIA UROLOGIAE EUROPAEAE

VOL. 17

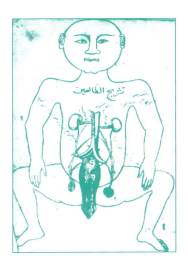

Edited by
Prof. Dr. Dirk Schultheiss

History Office
European Association of Urology
2010

The History Office of the EAU

D. Schultheiss (Chairman)	Giessen (DE)
C. Alamanis	Athens (GR)
J. Elo	Helsinki (FI)
R. Engel (AUA representative)	Linthicum, MD (US)
L.A. Fariña-Pérez	Madrid (ES)
J.F. Felderhof	The Hague (NL)
A. Figueiredo	Coimbra (PT)
P.P Figdor	Vienna (AT)
A. Jardin	Paris (FR)
J.J. Mattelaer	Kortrijk (BE)
S. Musitelli (Expert)	Zibidi San Giacomo (IT)
P. Rathert	Düsseldorf (DE)
I. Romics	Budapest (HU)
M. Skopec (Expert)	Vienna (AT)
R. Sosnowski	Warsaw (PL)
P. Thompson	London (UK)
A. Verit	Sanliurfa (TR)

CONTENTS of VOLUME 17
de Historia Urologiae Europaeae
(2010)

FOREWORD *by Per-Anders Abrahamsson*	7
INTRODUCTION *by Dirk Schultheiss*	11
THE 4th INTERNATIONAL CONGRESS ON THE HISTORY OF UROLOGY *By Rainer Engel*	15
JAQUES-LOUIS REVERDIN (1842-1929): THE SURGEON AND THE NEEDLE *By Luis A. Fariña-Pérez*	25
A HISTORICAL REVIEW OF FOURNIER'S GANGRENE *By José Medina Polo, Ana González-Rivas Fernández, Ángel Tejido Sánchez and Óscar Leíva Galvis*	37
JOHN HUNTER'S UROLOGIC DRAWINGS *By Michael E. Moran*	49
PATTISON FASCIA: THE FORGOTTEN EPONYM? *By Dirk Schultheiss*	61
DO UNTO YOURSELF AS YOU WOULD DO TO OTHERS - SELF-EXPERIMENTATION IN UROLOGY *By Johanna Thomas, Omer Karim, Hanif Motiwala and Amrith Raj Rao*	75
HISTORY OF THE TERM PROSTATE *Franz Josef Marx and Axel Karenberg*	89
ANDREAS VESALIUS AND SEMINAL ERRORS *By Michael E. Moran*	103

THE LEGEND OF SUN SHIMIAO: THE MAN WHO INVENTED URETHRAL CATHETERISATION **117**
By Wei Wang and Peter M. Thompson

THE "ORIENTAL TESTIS": A SHORT HISTORY **127**
By S.N. Cenk Buyukunal and Ayten Altıntaş

THE RELATIONSHIP BETWEEN THE PHYSICIAN AND THE INSTRUMENT MAKER **139**
By Michaela Zykan

TABLES OF CONTENTS VOLUMES 1-16 **151**

FOREWORD

At the beginning of each year I eagerly look forward to the documents collected and sent by our colleagues from the EAU History Office. To be invited to write the foreword has always been a pleasure since I get the first "crack" or glimpse at the contents of the newest edition in the *Historia* series before it goes to press.

The narratives of scientific query, the obstacles encountered by medical pioneers and how they were resolved by creative and resolute minds are unfailing sources of reading pleasure. The reflective essays and insightful accounts of the breakthroughs in medicine do not only inform us of the questions that vexed our predecessors, but also provide a succinct reminder that medicine is in a constant flux of renewal and change and that the practice and progress of our speciality are often closely linked to other spheres in human activity.

In this 17th edition of *Historia* one sees, for instance, the parallels between the world we live in today with that of the ancient Egyptians, or the early Ottoman Empire 800 years ago, when medical practitioners wrestled with the issue of castration, a practice considered taboo or illegal and yet practised illicitly or even condoned by the upper class and the ruling elite. Authors S.N. Cenk Buyukunal and Ayten Altıntaş traced the practice of castration in the Oriental world and clearly, as in our times, religious and political pressures have dictated heavily in the way medical investigators conducted their inquiry.

The spirit of discovery, however, proved to be irrepressible if not resilient. This same spirit is exemplified by Jaques-Louis Reverdin who founded modern Swiss surgery and is remembered for the first human transplant (skin grafting) and for designing the Reverdin needle, modifications of which are now used in modern laparoscopic surgery. Reverdin also possessed the quintessential European mind as he travelled across the continent's borders to share not only his innovations but also actively engaged his contemporaries in addressing the medical dilemmas they faced.

The quest of the European to push the boundaries of medicine is clearly demonstrated in the achievements of John Hunter (1728-1793) who left a lasting legacy in his collected works on anatomy and genitourinary illustrations. Belgian-born Andreas Vesalius (1514-1565) also earned a monumental place in medicine by placing anatomy and surgery back within the realm of science. In the article by J. Thomas and colleagues, the passion of the finest medical scientists even pushed them to self-experimentation, providing unassailable proof that to confront a challenge often requires personal sacrifice.

These are only a few of the fascinating narratives and descriptions of the epic journeys undertaken by the great minds in medicine and collected in this latest *Historia* edition. The *Historia* series do not only give recognition and credit to all those who paved the way before us, but also reaffirms the reality that progress in medicine is built on collective efforts and solidly sustained by those who are willing to question and make that leap necessary to bridge the gaps in our knowledge.

As in previous editions we are again impressed by and thankful for the dedication of our History Office, the authors and our editors to pursue this annual publishing project. And we hope that as you open and leaf through this book you will also share with us and rekindle the same creative spirit that inspired and has led to so many fascinating discoveries in the past.

PER-ANDERS ABRAHAMSSON
Secretary General EAU

INTRODUCTION

De Historia Urologiae Europaeae is a unique series. For almost two decades now, its readers have had an opportunity to look into the origins of urological knowledge in Europe and beyond its borders, to observe the history of our speciality as it unwraps and to enjoy the results of fascinating historical research.

This particular, 17th volume of *De Historia* stands out as special. Its publication is dedicated to the 25th Anniversary EAU Congress in Barcelona, the history of which to a large extent reflects the development of modern and cross-border European urology. The Congress has always been successful in building upon the achievements of the past and embracing the trends of the future - from subspecialisation to multidisciplinarity and internalisation. The meeting's unfailing companion, *De Historia*, mirrors and re-evaluates many of these developments from a historical perspective.

The 25th Anniversary of the EAU Congress is a milestone and a perfect opportunity to introduce symbolic changes into *De Historia*. It is now a modern-looking, beautifully type-set edition with interesting new solutions and room for creativity. The format has remained unchanged and the 17th volume will look perfectly good on your shelf with the rest of the series!

In this volume you will find an exciting constellation of articles by a truly international ensemble of authors. It is inspiring and encouraging to see that *De Historia* can rely on the commitment of talented professionals and enthusiastic urology historians, regardless of where they are based - the United States, Austria or China.

I am thankful to have had the help and the support of the EAU Central Office staff, E. Starkova and J. Vega; and I would like to extend a special thank you to the reviewers of the volume, P. M. Thompson, M. Skopec, S. Musitelli, R. Engel, A. Jardin, J. J. Mattelaer and A. Figueiredo, for their time, dedication and valuable commentary.

DIRK SCHULTHEISS
Chairman History Office EAU

THE 4TH INTERNATIONAL CONGRESS ON THE HISTORY OF UROLOGY

Rainer Engel

Expert History Office EAU, Curator William P. Didusch Center, Linthicum, USA.

The 4th International Congress on the History of Urology was held on 6-9 November, 2008 in Linthicum, Maryland, USA, where the headquarters of the American Urological Association are located. This was the first Congress on the History of Urology to be held outside of Europe. The meeting, sponsored by the AUA and supported by the EAU, drew 97 registered attendees from 11 countries in Europe and the United States. The meeting venue inside the AUA Headquarters was The William P. Didusch Center for Urologic History.

Dr. William Gee, Treasurer of the American Urological Association, opened the Congress by giving a summary of the history of the present modern building in which the Association is housed. Preceding the move to Linthicum, the AUA Headquarters was in downtown Baltimore, gradually expanding in size and number of employees from the initial single rowhouse that had been part of the estate of Hugh Hampton Young and four employees- to four townhouses cobbled together and over 100 employees.

Clearly the association was growing to a level that would no longer fit into this space. The decision was made to purchase land outside of town and in 2003 the new building was finished and occupied by association employees. Dr. Gee also talked about what is housed in

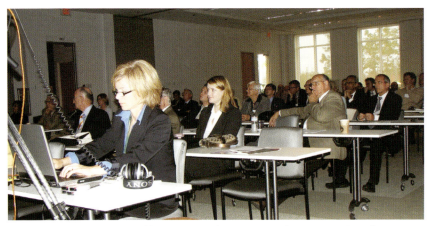

Figure 1: Participants of the 4th International Congress on the History of Urology at AUA Headquarters in Linthicum, Maryland, USA.

this building of 80,000 square feet. The museum occupies a significant part of the ground floor, which also includes a large conference and meeting room. Other floors house departments of Finance, Meetings, Industry Relations, Committee and Society Affairs, International, Marketing, Education, Health Policy, Research, and the AUA Foundation for patient education. At the date of this writing, the AUA has 140 employees.

Attendees heard fascinating presentations by medical students, urology residents, retired urologists, practicing urologists, as well as international experts such as Drs. Ralph Clayman, Alan Partin, Christian Chaussy, and Irwin Goldstein. They were treated to a stunning cross-section of where the specialty has been, how it developed, where urology is now, and were given some glimpses of the future. Prof. Frans Debruyne, past Secretary General of the EAU, gave an encapsulated history of the founding and subsequent growth of the European Urological Association.

We heard how serendipity led to the development of sildenafil citrate as an oral therapy for ED (Irv Goldstein). Eric Kouba mentioned how perseverance resulted in the development of radiology, and Christian Chaussy shared his experience in the conception and birth of ESWL and the resulting demise of the flank incision for kidney stones. Dr. Ralph Clayman took us back to the days when he and his team expanded laparoscopic surgery to new urological approaches.

These presentations made it quite clear that each of these discoveries was not the work of a single person but, as most events, took the creative force and collaboration of many to achieve what has resulted in today's urological armamentarium. We were treated to the history of the Storz Company by Dr. Matthias Reuter and an overview of the collaborative work between instrument maker and physician over the last 200 years by Michaela Zykan, Vienna. Pat Hanson presented the history of the American Cystoscope Makers, Inc. The most stirring presentation was given by Sakti Das, Historian of the AUA, on Marion Sims and his vesico-vaginal fistula experiments on black slaves, giving tribute to those women.

The Congress also took us on three site visits. We went downtown to tour The Johns Hopkins Hospital, where attendees learned how John Shaw Billings, an Army surgeon during the American Civil War, conceived not only the layout and design of the hospital buildings

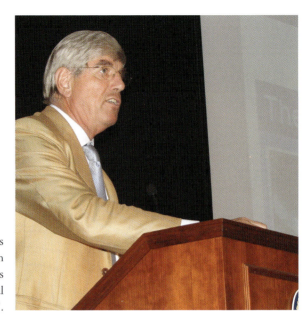

Figure 2: Prof. Frans Debruyne presents on "Famous Politicians and Their Urological Diseases".

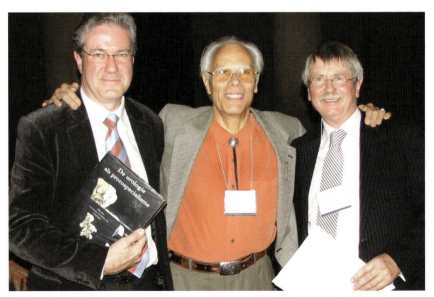

Figure 3: Dr. Rainer Engel (center) poses with Drs. Pelger and Felderhof from the Netherlands.

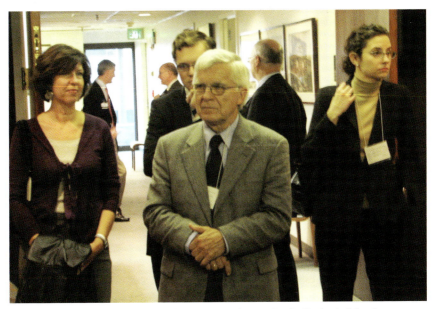

Figure 4: Congress attendees tour the James Buchanan Brady Urological Institute at Johns Hopkins Hospital in Baltimore, Maryland, USA.

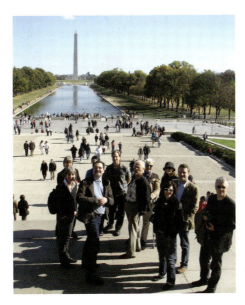

Figure 5: Congress attendees take in the sights of Washington, D.C., USA.

but also greatly expanded the vision of Johns Hopkins, the founder of this institution.

While Hopkins envisioned the hospital primarily as a resource for "the people of Baltimore," Billings went further, stating it should not be just a hospital for people of the area or even just for the United States but for people all over the world. Billings was also the visionary who felt that combining patient care, teaching, and research under one roof would create a unique facility. In those days it was indeed the only institution to do so.

Attendees then visited the Baltimore Museum of Art, which owes its existence and location to the vision and influence of Hugh Hampton Young, the first professor of urology at Hopkins who is also considered to be "The Father of American Urology." The museum is located on a parcel of land that used to be part of the property of Johns Hopkins University; it is known for its collection of relatively modern art. It contains all the art collected by the two Cone sisters, one of whom was an internist who had trained at Johns Hopkins and bequeathed her entire collection to this new museum. The Baltimore Museum of Art houses the largest collection of Matisse paintings, collected by Dr. Claribel Cone.

Funded by the American Urological Association and supported by a grant from Gyrus/ACMI, an Olympus Company, the Congress was a wonderful gathering of men and women who are interested in the preservation of our history, the lessons we can learn from the past, and the impact that history can have on future developments.

As one of the speakers, Professor F. J. Marx, wrote at the conclusion of the Congress, "This Congress had a very special character: mutual acceptance, a broad spectrum of stimulating presentations, a perfect and flexible organisation, and the unique ambiance of the museum created a warm, friendly and almost familiar atmosphere of international communication."

We all look forward to the next International Congress, hoping to be enriched by the presentations.

Correspondence to:
Rainer Engel
William P. Didusch Center for Urologic History
1000 Corporate Blvd
Linthicum, MD 21090, USA
E-mail: tstevens@auanet.org

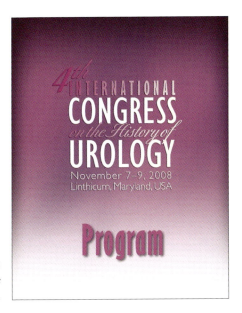

Figure 6: Cover of the programme book.

SPEAKER	PRESENTATION
Alan Partin	History of the Clinical Use And Misuse of PSA in Urology
Arthur Burnett	Highlights of Nitric Oxide Research
Ralph V. Clayman	Notes from the Lunatic Fringe: Musings on the First Laparoscopic Nephrectomy
Irwin Goldstein	History of Viagra
Pat Hanson	History of ACMI
Ajay Nehra	Surgery in Male Sexual Dysfunction
Peter Rathert	Benjamin Franklin (1706-1790) - His Relation to and Inventions for Urology and Medicine
Trinity Bivalacqua	Impotence and Priapism in the Ancient Times
Brian R. Matlaga	The Life and Works of Alexander Randall
Rainer M. Engel	Informed Consent
Sakti Das	Vesico-Vaginal Fistula Management - a Tribute to Anarcha, Betsy, Lucy and the Hamlins
Per-Anders Abrahamsson	Famous politicians and their urological diseases
Dirk Schultheiss	Sexuality History
Johan Mattelaer	Greco-Roman Phallic Culture in Medieval Western Europe
Frans Debruyne	The European Association of Urology (EAU)
Franz Josef Marx	A Confusing Story: The Prostate and Its Name
Fritz Moll	Votive Offerings, Devotional Objects and Souvenirs
Matthias Reuter	History of the Storz Company
Michaela Zykan	Instrument Maker and Physician: 200 Years of Endoscopy
Norberto Miguel Fredotovich	Germany: Physicians of Urology in Argentina
Christian Chaussy	History of ESWL
Lawrence Jones	History of Histories

Michael Moran	John Hunter's Urologic Drawings
Elise Halajian	Arpad Gerster and the Implementation of Photography
Genevieve Kruger	Contribution of Ramon Guiteras Toward Prostatectomy
Sutchin Patel	Denis Browne: Contributions to Pediatric Urology
Imre Romics	Medical Aid During the Revolution and War 1956
Bob Greenspan	Art of Collecting and Displaying Antique Surgical Instruments
George Drach	Shock Wave Lithotripsy: Problems with Intial FDA Studies
Lawrence Wyner	Peyronie and the Edict of 1743
Steven Selman	Photodynamic Diagnosis and Therapy
Erwin Rugendorff	Currency and Medicine
Sandra Moss	Common Sense for the Common (Wo) Man
Erik Kouba	Thomas Edison and the X-ray
Nicole Miller	The Oneida Experiment: "Male Continence" and Stirpiculture
Jennifer B. Gordetsky	The "Infertility" of Catherine de Medici and its Influence on 16th century France
Amrith Raj Rao	Encyclopaedia of the Images on the Art of Uroscopy
Johanna Thomas	Leonardo da Vinci and His Contribution to Medicine and Urology
Robert Donohue	George. E. Goodfellow, MD: Perineal Prostatectomist, Gunfighter's Surgeon, Linguist
William Parry	The Legacy of Dr. Richards P. Lyon
Daniel Fass	The History of Prostate Brachytherapy
Seshadri Sriprasad	"Vasectomania"
MA Omar	'Bladder stones' - the Catalyst for Advancement in Medical Science
Jennifer Hill	Horny Goats And Casanova: A Brief History Of The Aphrodisiac

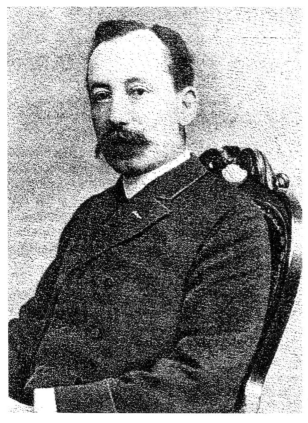

Figure 1:
Jaques-Louis Reverdin
as a young doctor.

JAQUES-LOUIS REVERDIN (1842-1929): THE SURGEON AND THE NEEDLE

Luis A. Fariña-Pérez

Member History Office EAU, Hospital Povisa, Vigo, Spain.

The development of abdominal laparoscopic techniques sparked the revival of the old Reverdin needle. It proved to be useful for the endoscopic closure of laparoscopic access ports, enabling to lower the incidence of incisional hernias[1]. Several new closing systems are in the market now, but most of them are modifications of the Reverdin needle with different names[2]. The new use of the old instrument prompted this review of the life and work of Jaques-Louis Reverdin, the Swiss surgeon who was educated in Paris and who played an instrumental role in the establishment of the modern surgery in Switzerland (Fig. 1).

1
Fariña-Pérez, L.A., Zungri, Telo E. "Cierre de los accesos laparoscópicos con la aguja de Reverdin: un nuevo uso para un viejo instrumento". *Actas Urol Esp.* 2003. 27:168-169.

2
Shaher, Z. "Port closure techniques". *Surg Endosc.* 2007. 21:1264-1274.

Training in Paris

Jaques-Louis Reverdin was born in Geneva, Switzerland, in 1842. He did his medical studies in Paris from 1862 to 1872. Very early in his training, from 1865, he started to practise in several well-known hospitals as *intern des hôpitaux et hospices civils*, in the role of a resident, so to speak. The Paris Hospital had already had its days of glory as a world leader in the field of medicine and surgery and was by then surpassed by the excellent centres in Vienna and Berlin.

Nevertheless, Reverdin had the opportunity to practise with several of the greatest surgery masters of the time, such as Leon Athanase Gosselin (1815-1887) from Hôpital La Pitié, who followed Dupuytren as teacher of anatomic dissection, and who worked and published on anatomic studies with Denonvilliers; Louis Alphonse Guérin (1816-1895) from Hôpital Saint Louis, who was the first to apply the ideas of Pasteur about atmospheric germs, who had a major interest in urologic surgery and whose name is associated with a valve in the fossa navicularis of the penis. Reverdin also trained at Hôpital Lariboisière and eventually, from 1869, at Hôpital Necker with Felix Guyon (1831-1920), the master and father of French urology. He completed his laboratory training with Louis A. Ranvier, the histologist who also inspired the work of Joaquin Albarrán on renal infections several years later[3].

[3] Reverdin, H. Jaques-Louis Reverdin (1842-1929). Un chirurgien à l'aube d'une ère nouvelle. Verlag Sauerländer: Aarau, Switzerland, 1971.

In 1869, while working with Prof. Guyon, he published on the pioneering experience of his successful free skin graft procedure for wound healing. He also presented the results at several meetings. The case was that of a 35-year-old man with an elbow injury from a fall. The skin in the area of the elbow was severely damaged and underwent complete necrosis. Reverdin removed two small slivers of epidermis from the right arm of the patient with a lancet, and placed them in the middle of the wound. Three days after he repeated the procedure and two weeks after, the implants had united covering the wound with a pale white plaque[4]. This work was an important milestone in plastic surgery - constituting the first organ transplantation ever and it immediately received world recognition[5]. Claude Bernard, a famous physiologist, commented on this breakthrough technology, which, in some cases, is still performed today and is known as the Reverdin graft, pinch or punch grafting[6].

[4] Reverdin, J.L. "Greffe epidermique-Experience faite dans le service de M. le docteur Guyon, à l'hôpital Necker". Bull Soc Imp de Chir de Paris. 1869. 10:511-515. Reprinted in: Plast Reconstr Surg. 1968. 41:79-82.

[5] Chick, L.R. "Brief history and biology of skin grafting". Ann Plast Surg. 1988. 21:358-365.

[6] Thami, G.P., Singal, A., Bhalla, M. "Surgical pearl: Full-thickness punch grafting in chronic non-healing ulcers". J Am Acad Dermatol. 2004. 50:99-100.

Reverdin was a superb medical student. In 1869, in his fourth year as intern, he was awarded the "gold medal of the Paris Hospital", a much appreciated prize for doctors in training. A year later, during the Paris siege by the Prussian army led by Otto von Bismarck, he took care of the injured people from the Swiss colony. By doing so, he took the advice of Ambroise Paré: "He who would be a surgeon should find an army and follow it." With that experience, some years later, he could teach military surgery to the Swiss military doctors and write a book *Leçons de chirurgie de guerre; des blessures par balles des fusils* (1910). After more than one year as a faculty member in Hôpital Necker, in 1870, he presented his doctoral thesis *Etude sur l'uréthrotomie interne* detailing carefully the experience of his master Guyon (63 operations, no deaths), gaining the valuable Civiale prize and the bronze medal of the Paris Faculty of Medicine.

His conclusions emphasised that the success of this blind approach to the treatment of the urethral disease was based on a careful indication, the mastering of the operation and the postoperative care of the patient. At that time, stenoses of the urethra was usually treated by dilation or external urethrotomy. Internal urethrotomy, performed with early instruments such as those used by Jean Civiale and Francois Guillon, was considered highly controversial.

Travelling through Europe
Following the success of his graft procedure, Reverdin embarked on a tour of foreign studies, travelling to Milan, London, Vienna and Berlin. He visited Billroth in Vienna, and

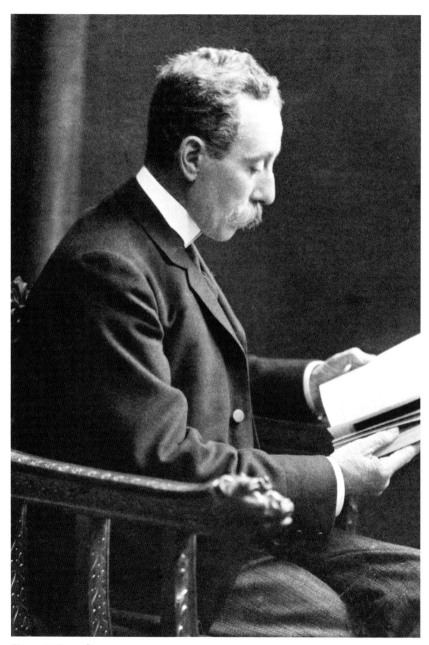
Figure 2: Reverdin as a senior surgeon.

Thomas Spencer Wells, who was known for his ovariectomies, in London. Thereafter he said that for the first time he could see patients not only operated on but also cured after these operations. This implies that only few patients survived after complicated abdominal operations in Paris. In those days, surgery was associated with high mortality due to pain, shock and septicaemia.

It was not until 1867 that Lister published in *The Lancet* his paper on antiseptic principles for surgical practice (immerse hands in antiseptic solution, treat instruments, gauzes and catgut with phenol solution prior to surgery). Lister's recommendations, and those of Louis Pasteur made a complete change in the until then cruel destiny of surgical patients. All of his life Reverdin was a supporter of Lister and Pasteur theories of antisepsis in surgery and he also wrote some papers on anaesthesia with ether in surgery. He preferred ether to chloroform, because the latter was difficult to administer; furthermore, the incorrect dosage often resulted in the death of the patients[3]. Not only pain, but also fever almost disappeared from the natural evolution of the operated patient.

Return to Geneva

He returned back to Geneva in 1872 to begin a long surgical practice in the cantonal hospital and in his private clinic, which he co-founded with his cousin Auguste Reverdin[7]. He also taught at the University of Geneva (where a Faculty of Medicine was created in 1876) between 1876 and 1910. He taught on external operative pathology, including pathology of male urinary and genital organs (Fig. 2).

[7] Saudan, G. "Jaques-Louis Reverdin (1842-1929) et son cousin Auguste (1848-1908). Ou quand la clinique chirurgicale précède la physiologie expérimentale". *Rev Méd Suisse Romande*. 1993. 113:567-581.

The Reverdin needle and other contributions

He made several contributions to the study of thyroid diseases, which were highly prevalent in Geneva and the neighbouring regions, in particular on functional deficiency following total or partial removal of the thyroid gland (postoperative myxoedema or cachexia strumipriva), in 1882.

In a beautifully illustrated paper, which he presented with his cousin Auguste Reverdin, he remarked that in this operation "...[he] respects the enveloping membrane, or preserves a part of [thyroid] gland". These observations were made at the same time by Theodor Kocher in Bern, and there was a long dispute between Reverdin and Kocher on who was the first to describe the endocrine function of the thyroid, something that contributed so much to the foundation of endocrinology as a science. In the end it was Kocher, having performed over 5000 thyroid operations in his lifetime, who received in solitary the Nobel Prize for these studies in 1909.

Reverdin was also interested in and wrote papers on genitourinary problems (urethrotomy, penile fistula, bladder trauma, tuberculosis cystitis, prostatitis, vesicovaginal fistula and urethrorectal fistula). He collaborated with his two friends and colleagues from the Paris times, Jean-Louis Prevost, who was a doctor with an orientation to neurology and physiology, and Constant Picot, who was a general practitioner and historian; all three of them were interns at various Paris hospitals and doctors at the University of Paris. In 1880 they founded the *Revue Medicale de la Suisse Romande*, the most

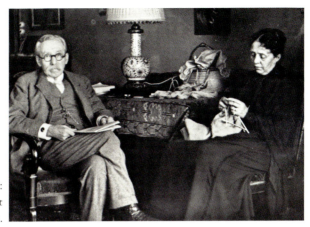

Figure 3: Reverdin retired, at home with his wife.

[8] Mayer, R. "Ils étaient trois!. Jaques-Louis Reverdin, Jean-Louis Prevost et Constant Picot, fondateurs de la Revue médicale de la Suisse romande. Evocation de la naissance d'une revue médicale et esquisse biographique de ses premiers rédacteurs". Rev Méd Suisse Romande. 1980. 100:1013-1041.

[9] Kirkup, J. "The history and evolution of surgical instruments. V. Needles and their penetrating derivatives". Ann Roy Coll Surg Engl. 1986. 68:29-33.

important Swiss medical journal of the late 19th century and the whole 20th century, which was discontinued in 2004[8].

Reverdin retired in 1910 and dedicated himself to the study of butterflies, making important naturalistic studies for the following 18 years (Fig. 3). He was a founding member and president of the Lepidopterologic Society of Geneva, wrote some 45 papers on the classification and characteristics of several species of butterflies and gave his collections of butterflies, his books on the subject and more than 10.000 microscopic preparations of his studies to the Natural History Museum. He died in 1929 at the age of 86.

Reverdin is particularly remembered in the field of surgery and urology for a special needle driver that he created in 1879. The needle had a slot eye controlled by a lever used to pass a suture to control organ pedicles and vessels. This was a significant breakthrough in the time when catgut and silk were the most employed sutures[9]. This needle is a modification

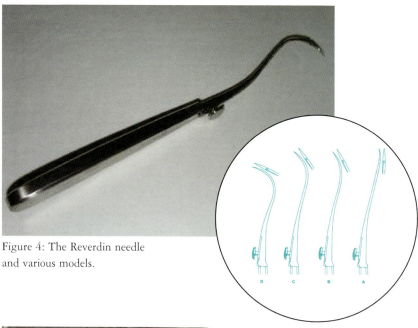

Figure 4: The Reverdin needle and various models.

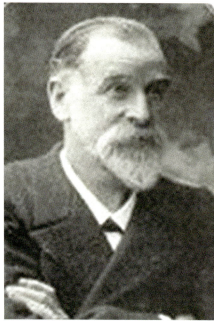

Figure 5: Dr. Lucas Championnière, who introduced Listerian principles of antiseptic surgery in France and wrote the first book on the topic (*Chirurgie antiseptic*, 1880), which was translated into English under the title *Antiseptic surgery: The principles, modes of application, and results of the Lister dressing*, 1881.

with substantial improvement of some preceding models such as the Deschamps needle manufactured by Charrière, and that of the German surgeon Victor von Bruns.

The Reverdin needle was manufactured by the Swiss instrument maker Felix Demaurex. Later on, it was modified by his cousin August Reverdin (1848-1908) and nephew Albert Reverdin (1881-1929), and manufactured by the best instrument makers in different angles and forms, enabling the operator to perform sutures either in profound or superficial surgical fields (Fig. 4).

Dr. J. Lucas Championnière (Fig. 5), a French colleague and friend of Reverdin, said the following about this needle, in 1910:

> After you returned to Geneva, you invented a needle to which not enough praise has been given. I love it, not only because I appreciate it for having employed it all my life, but above all because every day it reminds me about the careful, meticulous, precise and practical comrade. I have used it in all its forms, I have had big ones, small ones, right ones, curve ones, and having needed a soft needle, I've made one of your model[3].

Nowadays, with the development and rise of abdominal laparoscopic techniques, the old Reverdin needle enjoys a revival, being effectively used for the closure of laparoscopic access ports[2].

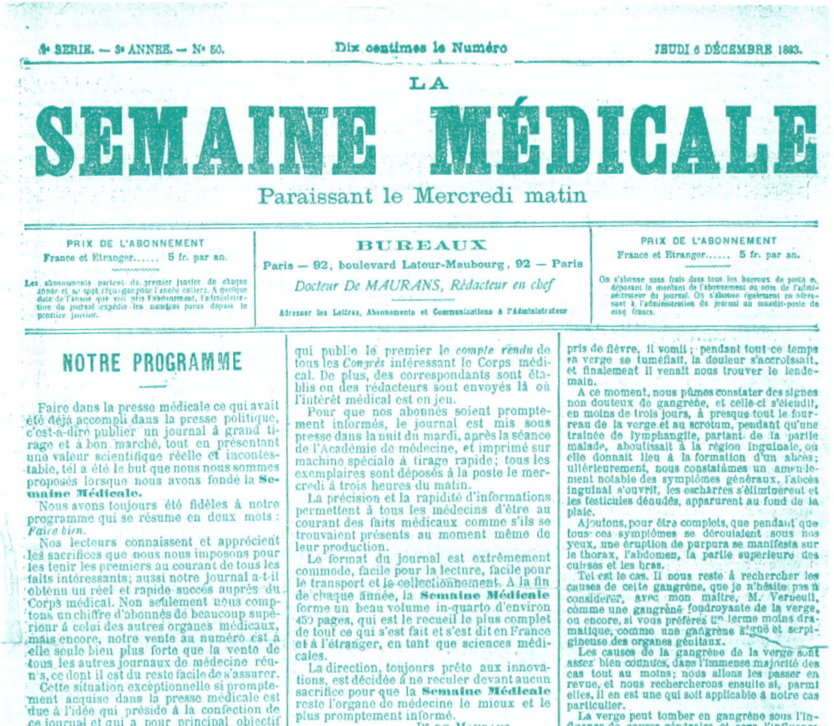

4e SÉRIE. — 3e ANNÉE. — N° 50. Dix centimes le Numéro JEUDI 6 DÉCEMBRE 1883.

LA

SEMAINE MÉDICALE

Paraissant le Mercredi matin

PRIX DE L'ABONNEMENT

France et Étranger...... 5 fr. par an.

Les abonnements partent du premier janvier de chaque année et ne sont reçus que pour l'année entière. A quelque date de l'année que soit pris l'abonnement, l'administration du journal expédie les numéros parus depuis le premier janvier.

BUREAUX

Paris — 92, boulevard Latour-Maubourg, 92 — Paris

Docteur De MAURANS, Rédacteur en chef

Adresser les Lettres, Abonnements et Communications à l'Administrateur

PRIX DE L'ABONNEMENT

France et Étranger...... 5 fr. par an.

On s'abonne sans frais dans tous les bureaux de poste en déposant le montant de l'abonnement au nom de l'administrateur du journal. On s'abonne également en adressant à l'administration du journal un mandat-poste de cinq francs.

NOTRE PROGRAMME

Faire dans la presse médicale ce qui avait été déjà accompli dans la presse politique, c'est-à-dire publier un journal à grand tirage et à bon marché, tout en présentant une valeur scientifique réelle et incontestable, tel a été le but que nous nous sommes proposés lorsque nous avons fondé la **Semaine Médicale.**

Nous avons toujours été fidèles à notre programme qui se résume en deux mots : *Faire bien.*

Nos lecteurs connaissent et apprécient les sacrifices que nous nous imposons pour les tenir les premiers au courant de tous les faits intéressants; aussi notre journal a-t-il obtenu un réel et rapide succès auprès du Corps médical. Non seulement nous comptons un chiffre d'abonnés de beaucoup supérieur à celui des autres organes médicaux, mais encore, notre vente au numéro est à elle seule bien plus forte que la vente de tous les autres journaux de médecine réunis, ce dont il est du reste facile de s'assurer.

Cette situation exceptionnelle si promptement acquise dans la presse médicale est due à l'idée qui préside à la confection de ce journal et qui a pour principal objectif de donner l'événement de la semaine de la manière la plus complète et la plus immédiate.

D'ailleurs, il est suffisamment établi sans qu'il soit besoin de le démontrer ici, que la **Semaine Médicale** est bien un véritable journal et non une revue comme tous les autres journaux de médecine, qui s'attachent peu à publier à la première heure les faits que recherchent particulièrement nos reporters toujours en quête de la nouveauté médicale.

Outre les *Travaux originaux* et les *Revues* consacrés aux *diverses branches* de la *Science médicale*, à la *Presse française* et *étrangère*, aux *Intérêts professionnels*, à la *Pharmacie*, à la *Médecine vétérinaire*, etc., chaque numéro contient :

Une *leçon clinique* recueillie par la *sténographie* dans un des services de médecine ou de chirurgie des hôpitaux de Paris;

Le *compte rendu* exact et complet des *Sociétés savantes* ayant siégé pendant la semaine : Académie de médecine, Sociétés de chirurgie, de biologie, de médecine légale, Société médicale des hôpitaux, etc., etc.

On y trouve également le *compte rendu* des séances des deux principales Sociétés médicales de Berlin : la *Société de médecine berlinoise* et la *Société de médecine interne*. Ce compte rendu nous est fourni, en français, par notre correspondant spécial à Berlin, et la publication en est faite dans les mêmes conditions de fidélité et de célérité que nous observons à l'égard des Sociétés savantes de Paris.

La **Semaine Médicale** est le journal qui publie le premier le *compte rendu* de tous les *Congrès* intéressant le Corps médical. De plus, des correspondants sont établis ou des rédacteurs sont envoyés là où l'intérêt médical est en jeu.

Pour que nos abonnés soient promptement informés, le journal est mis sous presse dans la nuit du mardi, après la séance de l'Académie de médecine, et imprimé sur machine spéciale à tirage rapide; tous les exemplaires sont déposés à la poste le mercredi à trois heures du matin.

La précision et la rapidité d'informations permettent à tous les médecins d'être au courant des faits médicaux comme s'ils se trouvaient présents au moment même de leur production.

Le format du journal est extrêmement commode, facile pour la lecture, facile pour le transport et le collectionnement. A la fin de chaque année, la **Semaine Médicale** forme un beau volume in-quarto d'environ 450 pages, qui est le recueil le plus complet de tout ce qui s'est fait et s'est dit en France et à l'étranger, en tant que sciences médicales.

La direction, toujours prête aux innovations, est décidée à ne reculer devant aucun sacrifice pour que la **Semaine Médicale** reste l'organe de médecine le mieux et le plus promptement informé.

Dr DE MAURANS.

A partir de ce jour, les nouveaux abonnés pour l'année prochaine (1884) recevront gratuitement les numéros de la **Semaine Médicale** à paraître jusqu'au 31 décembre 1883.

En *France*, en *Algérie*, en *Suisse*, en *Italie*, en *Belgique*, en *Hollande*, en *Suède* et *Norvège*, en *Danemark* et en *Portugal*, on s'abonne sans frais dans tous les bureaux de poste. Il suffit de verser la somme de *cinq francs*, montant de l'abonnement annuel, que le bureau de poste se charge de faire parvenir à l'Administration du journal avec toutes les indications nécessaires.

On peut également s'abonner en adressant à l'Administration du journal un mandat-poste ou un bon de poste de cinq francs.

La **Semaine Médicale** entrera dans sa quatrième année le 1er janvier 1884.

CLINIQUE MÉDICALE

Hôpital Saint-Louis. — M. le professeur FOURNIER.

Gangrène foudroyante de la verge.

Vous venez d'assister, dans nos salles, à un triste spectacle; il s'agit d'un homme, jeune encore, dont les organes génitaux externes tombent en gangrène.

Le vendredi 16, cet homme se levait en bonne santé et allait à l'atelier où il est mouleur en cuivre. Quelque temps après, il éprouvait une légère douleur à la verge, et il constatait en même temps à ce niveau une petite rougeur. Il ne s'en inquiéta pas tout d'abord, mais la douleur devenant plus vive, il rentra chez lui vers trois heures et se coucha. A ce moment, il fut pris de fièvre, il vomit; pendant tout ce temps sa verge se tuméfiait, la douleur s'accroissait, et finalement il venait nous trouver le lendemain.

A ce moment, nous pûmes constater des signes non douteux de gangrène, et celle-ci s'étendit, en moins de trois jours, à presque tout le fourreau de la verge et au scrotum, pendant qu'une traînée de lymphangite, partant de la partie malade, aboutissait à la région inguinale, où elle donnait lieu à la formation d'un abcès; ultérieurement, nous constatâmes un amendement notable des symptômes généraux, l'abcès inguinal s'ouvrit, les eschares s'éliminèrent et les testicules dénudés, apparurent au fond de la plaie.

Ajoutons, pour être complets, que pendant que tous ces symptômes se déroulaient sous nos yeux, une éruption de purpura se manifesta sur le thorax, l'abdomen, la partie supérieure des cuisses et les bras.

Tel est le cas. Il nous reste à rechercher les causes de cette gangrène, que je n'hésite pas à considérer, avec mon maître, M. Verneuil, comme une gangrène foudroyante de la verge, ou encore, si vous préférez un terme moins dramatique, comme une gangrène aiguë et serpigineuse des organes génitaux.

Les causes de la gangrène de la verge sont assez bien connues, dans l'immense majorité des cas tout au moins; nous allons les passer en revue, et nous rechercherons ensuite si, parmi elles, il en est une qui soit applicable à notre cas particulier.

La verge peut tomber en gangrène sous l'influence de causes générales, et sous l'influence de causes locales, ces dernières s'observant bien plus fréquemment que les premières.

Parmi les causes générales, une des plus importantes est le diabète, dont l'influence a été signalée, il y a longtemps déjà, par Marchal de Calvi. Il est vrai que c'est surtout sur les membres que le diabète porte le plus habituellement son action destructive; mais la verge est bien loin d'être à l'abri d'une pareille manifestation.

Le sphacèle porte parfois sur la verge en même temps que sur d'autres régions du corps. Il me souvient d'avoir vu un malade dans ces conditions; j'avais constaté sur sa verge une plaque blanche diphthéroïde, de l'étendue d'une pièce d'un franc, que je ne savais à quoi attribuer, lorsque j'appris fortuitement que le malade était diabétique. Mon attention ayant été mise en éveil par cette révélation, j'examinai le reste de son corps, et je ne tardai pas à y découvrir une série d'exanthèmes, qui ne pouvaient laisser aucun doute sur la nature du mal.

D'autres fois, la gangrène diabétique porte exclusivement sur la verge, et dans ce cas, elle est le plus souvent causée par un traumatisme. Les diabétiques, on l'a dit avec raison, sont de véritables *noli me tangere*, la moindre plaie, l'opération chirurgicale la plus anodine par elle-même, peut être pour eux l'occasion de véritables complications. A l'appui de mon dire, il me serait facile de vous citer un grand nombre de gangrènes de la verge succédant à l'opération de la circoncision.

Un bel exemple du genre a été publié par M. de Beauvais.

Il s'agissait d'un homme de trente-quatre ans atteint d'un phimosis compliqué de balano-posthite. On l'opère; les deux jours qui suivent l'opération ne présentent rien d'insolite, mais le troisième, survient une hémorrhagie abondante, le cinquième, la plaie prend l'aspect d'un phlegmon gangréneux, et ce dernier se propage à toute

Figure 1: *"Gangrène foudroyante de la verge"* by Jean Alfred Fournier, *La Semaine Médicale*. 1883. By courtesy of the Bibliothèque Interuniversitaire de Médecine, Paris.

HISTORICAL REVIEW OF FOURNIER`S GANGRENE: BAURIENNE, 1764, AND HEROD THE GREAT, 4 B.C.

José Medina Polo,
Ana González-Rivas Fernández,
Ángel Tejido Sánchez,
Óscar Leíva Galvis

Hospital Universitario 12 de Octubre, Department of Urology, Madrid, Spain.

Complutense University of Madrid, Department of Classical Philology, Madrid, Spain.

1
Fournier, J.A. "Gangrène foudroyante de la verge". *Sem Med.* 1883. 3:345-347.

2
Corman, M.L., editor. "Classic Articles in colonic and rectal surgery: Jean-Alfred Fournier 1832-1914". *Dis Colon Rectum.* 1988. 31:984-8.

3
Baurienne, H. "Sur une plaie contuse qui s'est terminée pour la sphacele de le scrotum". *J Med Chir Pharm.* 1764. 20:251-256.

4
Hirschmann, J.V., Richardson, P., Kramer, R.S., Mackowiak, P.A. "Death of an Arabian Jew". *Arch Inter Med.* 2004. 164:833-839.

In 1883, Jean Alfred Fournier described a necrotising fasciitis of the genital area, which is nowadays known as Fournier's gangrene (Figs. 1, 2). This genital gangrene possesses certain specific characteristics:
1. The absence of any obvious cause
2. Specific symptoms, principally:
   a. a sudden onset of gangrene;
   b. an astonishingly rapid spread of this gangrene, always considerable in extent;
   c. the frequent coexistence of purple discoloration;
   d. a high rate of mortality[1, 2].

However, some genital gangrenes described before Fournier's report are nowadays also often considered to be Fournier's gangrene, and two of these cases are the object of our attention here. In 1764, for example, Baurienne described a necrotising fasciitis of the genital region[3]; and, based on the description of Flavius Josephus, the cause of death of Herod the Great could also have been kidney failure complicated by Fournier's gangrene[4].

The purpose of this study is to re-examine these cases.

Figure 2: *"Gangrène foudroyante de la verge"* by Jean Alfred Fournier, *La Semaine Médicale* 1883. By courtesy of the Bibliothèque Interuniversitaire de Médecine, Paris.

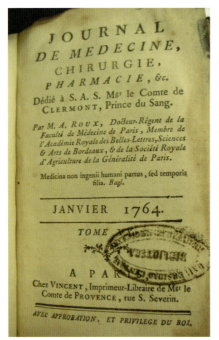

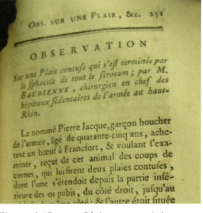

Figure 4: *"Sur une Plaie contuse qui s'est terminée par le sphacele de tout le scrotum"* by Baurienne, *Journal de Médecine, Chirurgie, Pharmacie, &C.* 1764. By courtesy of the Historical Library Marqués de Valdecilla (UCM).

Figure 3: *Journal de Médecine, Chirurgie, Pharmacie, &C.* 1764. By courtesy of the Historical Library Marqués de Valdecilla (UCM).

Baurienne, 1764

Baurienne reported a case of scrotal gangrene in the *Journal de Medecine, Chirurgie, Pharmacie, &C*. The article was titled *"Sur une Plaie contuse qui s'est terminée par le sphacele de tout le scrotum"*[3] and it is considered to be the first case of Fournier gangrene published in literature[5,6] (Figs. 3, 4).

We have reviewed and analysed this case of scrotal gangrene using a copy of the article from the Historical Library Marqués de Valdecilla at the Complutense University of Madrid.

Baurienne highlighted the case of a 45-year-old man, an army butcher, who was given medical attention four days after suffering an injury in the genital region and the left thigh. This injury was caused by the horns of an ox.

The patient was suffering from fever and abdominal distension, and had difficulty speaking. The genital area was affected by gangrene, which spread from the right lower edge of the pubic bone to the perineum, and the left testicle was devitalised; it seemingly was not receiving irrigation.

First of all, the patient was revived, and then surgery was performed and the necrotising tissues removed. The wound was left open, covered by gauzes impregnated with oxygenated water, and was dressed daily. For a few days, the patient's condition seemed to improve, but the gangrene returned once more, and another surgical intervention was required. The whole scrotal area was affected by gangrene, so an

---

[5] Paty, R., Smith, A.D. "Gangrene and Fournier's gangrene". *Urol Clin North Am.* 1992. 19:149-162.

[6] Smith, G.L., Bunker, C.B., Dinneen, M.D. "Fournier's gangrene". *Br J Urol.* 1998. 81:347-55.

> - *Flavius Josephus. Jewish Antiquities (AI, 17.169)*
>
>   ναὶ μὴν καὶ τοῦ αἰδοίου σῆψις σκώληκας ἐμποιοῦσα
>
>   "as well as for a gangrene of his privy parts that produced works"
>
> - *Flavius Josephus. The Jewish War (BI, 1.656)*
>
>   καὶ δὴ αἰδοίου σηπεδών σκώληκας γεννῶσα
>
>   "and gangrene of the privy parts, engendering worms"

Figure 5: Greek translation of *Jewish Antiquities* (IA, 17.169) and *The Jewish War* (BI, 1.656) by Flavius Josephus.

aggressive surgical debridement was performed and all necrotic tissues resected. The left scrotal wall too was resected, so that the left testicle remained exposed: *"le teſticule gauche ſe trouva à découvert, & dépouillé de ſes tuniques communes"*. An orchiectomy was performed on the right side, because the right testicle had rotted, and the spermatic cord could not even be identified.

Despite the second operation, the patient did not improve, and the fever lasted for ten days. After this period, the fever disappeared, the patient began to get better, and the wound started to heal. New skin cells gradually covered the left testicle and within two months the patient was cured and the area re-epithelialised, but the scrotal area remained smaller and hairless: *"le teſticule gauche ſe recouvroit de chairs grenues et vermeilles."*

Baurienne concluded that in cases of scrotal gangrene, radical surgical debridement of all infected and necrotic tissues is required. However, the testicles are not always affected, and in these cases they must not be resected. As Baurienne stated, the preservation of the testicles is necessary to safeguard the male reproductive system:

> ...lorfqu'ils emportent un fcrotum entiérement fphacélé, de ne point emporter les tefticules qui fe trouvent fouvent confondus avec toutes les parties. Cette remarque eft de la derniere conféquence, puifque l'on priveroit un homme de fervir à la propagation de fon efpece.

Herod the Great

Some authors have suggested that the cause of death of Herod the Great was Fournier's gangrene[4]. Flavius Josephus described Herod's death in two different books: *The Jewish War (Bellum Iudaicum:* BI) and *Jewish Antiquities (Antiquitates Iudaicae:* AI)[7, 8]. In *Jewish Antiquities*, Flavius Josephus mentions that Herod the Great suffered "gangrene of his privy parts that produced worms" (AI, 17.169) (Fig. 5) This study has reviewed the literature published about Herod the Great's disease, including the description by Flavius Josephus in the Greek-English editions of *Jewish Antiquities* and of *The Jewish War*, translated respectively by Marcus (Loeb Classical Library, 1980)[8] and by Thackeray (Loeb Classical Library, 1989)[7].

Herod's disease was described by Flavius Josephus in both books as follows:

> But Herod's illness became more and more acute, for God was inflicting just punishment upon him for his lawless deeds. The fever that he had was a light one and did not so much indicate symptoms of inflammation to the touch as it

[7] Josephus, F. *Josephus in Nine Volumes. Vol. 2, The Jewish War (Bellum Iudaicum),* books I-III, translated into English by H. St. J. Thackeray, Cambridge (MASS). London: Loeb Classical Library, 1989.

[8] Josephus, F. *Josephus in Ten Volumes. Vol. 8, Jewish Antiquities (Antiquitates Iudaicae),* books XV-XVII, translated into English by R. Marcus. Cambridge (MASS). Loeb Classical Library: London, 1980.

produced internal damage. He also had a terrible desire to scratch himself because of this, for it was impossible not to seek relief. There was also an ulceration of the bowels and intestinal pains that were particularly terrible, and a moist, transparent suppuration of the feet. And he suffered similarly from an abdominal ailment, as well as from a gangrene of his privy parts that produced worms. His breathing was marked by extreme tension, and it was very unpleasant because of the disagreeable exhalation of his breath and his constant gasping. He also had convulsions in every limb that took on unendurable severity. Accordingly it was said by the men of God and by those whose special wisdom led them to proclaim their opinions on such matters that all this was penalty that God was exacting of the king for his great impiety (AI, 17.168-170).

From this time onwards Herod's malady began to spread to his whole body and his sufferings took a variety of forms. He had fever, though not a raging fever, an intolerable itching of the whole skin, continuous pains in the intestines, tumours in the feet as in dropsy, inflammation of the abdomen and gangrene of the privy parts, engendering worms, in addition to asthma, with great difficulty in breathing, and convulsions in all his limbs (BI, 1.656).

Many scholars have tried to identify Herod's disease[9, 10, 11]. If Josephus indeed provided an accurate and objective account, the list

[9] Sandison, A.T. "The last illness of Herod the Great, King of Judaea". *Med Hist*. 1967. 11(4):381-388.

[10] Ladouceur, D.J. "The Death of Herod the Great". *Classical Philology*. 1981. 76(1):25-34.

[11] Litchfield, W.R. "The bittersweet demise of Herod the Great". *J R Soc Med* 1998. 91(5):283-284.

of symptoms would indicate a chronic kidney disease complicated by Fournier's gangrene[5, 11]. Other scientists, however, have proposed diagnoses such as syphilis, cirrhosis of the liver, or diabetes mellitus. What is more, diabetes mellitus could be the aetiology behind the kidney failure[5, 12, 13, 14].

However, certain historical circumstances must be taken into account. On the one hand, Flavius Josephus and Herod were not contemporaries: Josephus was born about forty years after Herod's death. Nor were Josephus' works published at the same time: *The Jewish War* was published between 75 and 79 A.D., and *Jewish Antiquities* twenty years later. This interval of time also implies a change of perspective: in *Jewish Antiquities*, Josephus' attitude towards the Romans is more critical, as can be seen in the tone used. Finally, it is said that Josephus was influenced by the biography of Herod the Great written by Nicolaus of Damascus, who was a friend and historian of Herod, and the author of a universal history. However, these documents have been lost, so our knowledge of Nicolaus of Damascus' text is limited to indirect sources[4, 9].

Nicolaus of Damascus was one of Herod's most trusted advisors, and so it is probable that the tone used in his biography of Herod is a positive one. As some scholars have suggested, therefore, if Josephus' description is wholly based on details taken from Nicolaus of Damascus, then the negative points that Josephus made about Herod the Great are very probably true[4]. However, despite using Nicolaus' text as one of his main sources, Josephus criticises this work very severely.

12
Hollenberg, N.K. "Lead exposure and chronic renal failure". *Arch Inter Med.* 2004. 164:2507.

13
Madariaga, M.G., Smith, P.W. "Infectious disease consultation for Herod the Great". *Arch Inter Med.* 2004. 164:2507-2508.

14
Johnson, S.R. "Herod the Great and polyarteritis nodosa". *Arch Inter Med.* 2004. 164:2508.

Josephus was Jewish, and was hostile towards Herod, because the latter was considered a "half Jew": he was in fact Idumean, from a people who had adopted Jewish practices only two generations earlier. Herod was also named king of Judea by the Romans, and was therefore viewed as a Roman collaborator and a traitor to the faith and political independence of the Jews[9]. Moreover, Nicolaus of Damascus' work is not Josephus' only reference: some scholars have pointed out that the description of Herod's disease in the *Antiquities* imitates Thucydides' account of the Athenian plague in the *History of the Peloponnesian War*, written in the 5th century B.C.[10]:

> That year, as was agreed by all, happened to be unusually free from disease so far as regards the other maladies; but if anyone was already ill of any disease all terminate in this. In other cases from no obvious cause, but suddenly and while in good health, men were seized first with intense heat of the head, and redness and inflammation of the eyes, and the parts inside the mouth, both the throat and the tongue, immediately became blood-red and <u>exhaled an unnatural and fetid breath</u>. In the next stage sneezing and hoarseness came on, and in a short time the disorder descended to the chest, attended by severe coughing. And when it settled in the stomach, that was upset, and vomits of bile of every kind named by physicians ensued, they also attended by great distress; and in most cases ineffectual retching followed produced <u>violent convulsions</u>, which sometimes abat-

ed directly, sometimes not until long afterwards. Externally, the body was not so very warm to the touch; it was not pale, but reddish, livid, and breaking out in small blisters and ulcers. But internally it was consumed by such a heat that patients could not bear to have on them the lightest coverings or linen sheets, but wanted to be quite uncovered and would have liked best to throw themselves into cold water - indeed many of those who were not looked after did throw themselves into cisterns - so tormented were they by thirst which could not be quenched; and it was all the same whether they drunk much or little. They were also beset by restlessness and sleeplessness which never abated. And the body was not wasted while the disease was at its height, but resisted surprisingly the ravages of the disease, so that when the patient died, as most of them did on the seventh or ninth day from the internal heat, they still had some strength left; or, if they passed the crisis, the disease went down into the bowels, producing there a violent ulceration, and at the same time an acute diarrhoea set in, so that in the later stage most of them perished through weakness caused by it. For the malady, starting from the head where it was first seated, passed down until it spread through the whole body, and if one got over the worst, it seized upon the extremities at least and left its marks there, for it attacked the privates and fingers and toes, and many escaped with the loss of these, though some lost their eyes also. In some cases

Flavius Josephus - Herod the Great	Thucydides - The Athenian Plague
- Mild fever	- The body was not so very warm to the touch
- Disagreeable exhalation of his breath	- Exhaled an unnatural and fetid breath
- Ulcerations of the bowels and intestinal pains	- Went down into the bowels, producing there a violent ulceration
- Convulsions in every limb	- Violent convulsions
- Gangrene of the genitalia	- It attacked the privates

Table 1: Comparison between Josephus and Thucydides books.

the sufferer was attacked immediately after recovery by loss of memory, which extended to every object alike, so that the failed to recognize either themselves or their friends" (Th., 2.49)[15] (Table 1).

It should also be taken into account that the Jews of Josephus' time would typically relate medical symptoms to moral faults. Specific symptoms were the results of specific sins: ulcers, for instance, tended to be related to immorality and sexual offenses.[10,16] Throughout *Jewish Antiquities*, Josephus refers repeatedly to Herod's licentiousness and uncontrolled sexuality; it should be remembered that Herod had ten wives and that he lived in polygamy, which was a permissible, if rare, practice in ancient Judaism[9-11]. Moreover, Josephus emphasised the divine aetiology of Herod's disease, and this can be seen from the very beginning of the description of Herod's disease in *Jewish Antiquities*, when Josephus affirmed that "God was inflicting just punishment upon him for his lawless

[15] Thucydides. *History of the Peloponnesian War*. Vol. 2, books III-IV, translated into English by Charles Forster Smith, Cambridge (MASS)., Loeb Classical Library: London, 1975.

[16] Ladouceur, D.J. "The Language of Josephus". *Journal for the Study of Judaism in the Persian, Hellenistic and Roman Period*. 1983. 14:18-38.

deeds" (AI, 17.168) In short, it seems likely that Josephus' account was influenced by certain cultural beliefs that determined his description of Herod's disease[10].

Because of all the above evidence, it is our contention that Josephus' description of Herod's disease is not an objective one. Josephus used the text by Nicolaus of Damascus to write his life of Herod, but Josephus' purpose is to criticise Herod's behaviour and to show the punishment he received because of it. It is not therefore reasonable to base a diagnosis of Herod's affliction on an analysis of Josephus' list of symptoms, whether that diagnosis be Fournier's gangrene or any other illness.

Conclusions

Baurienne's article shows the management of the scrotal gangrene from the point of view of a surgeon. According to his conclusions, all affected tissues have to be removed, bearing in mind that the testicles are not frequently affected. However, the case described by Baurienne was the consequence of a previous trauma, so it was not an idiopathic case of Fournier's gangrene. On the other hand, it is probable that Josephus' description of Herod the Great's death over-emphasised his uncontrolled sexuality, and on that basis it also appears unlikely that he suffered from Fournier's gangrene. Our conclusion is, therefore, that neither of these cases can be established as the gangrene originally described by Fournier.

Acknowledgements

The authors of this paper wish to express their sincere gratitude for the support provided by the Historical Library Marqués de Valdecilla at Complutense University of Madrid and the Bibliothèque Interuniversitaire de Médecine in Paris.

Correspondence to:
José Medina Polo
Department of Urology
Hospital Universitario 12 de Octubre
Avda. de Andalucía s/n, 28041 Madrid, Spain
E-Mail: josemedinapolo@telefonica.net

JOHN HUNTER'S UROLOGIC DRAWINGS

Southwest Urology, Tucson, USA.

Michael E. Moran

[1]
Moore, W. *The Knife Man. Blood, Body Snatching, and the Birth of Modern Surgery.* Broadway Books: New York, 2005.

[2]
Paget, S. *John Hunter, Man of Science and Surgeon.* Fischer Unwin: London, 1897.

[3]
Hunter, J. "On the descent of the testis". In: Hunter, W. *Medical Commentaries.* A. Hamilton: London, 1762.

John Hunter was born the tenth and youngest child to a Scottish family in midwinter during the early hours of 14 February 1728[1]. His father was 65 when John was born, and they were never very close, his mother was indulgent and he developed his own sort of individualism. He detested formal lessons and classic reading. There is some evidence that John, in fact was dyslexic[1]. "I pestered people with questions about what nobody knew or cared anything about." His youth was centred upon his interest in nature and he was not interested in the formal education available at the time.

At the age of 20, he followed his older brother, William, to London to learn about anatomy. Under the tutelage of his gifted older brother, John quickly learned both human and comparative anatomy. Though beginning with dissection, he soon began teaching anatomy and making specimens for demonstration. With the help of his brother's influence, he managed to become a surgical pupil at St. Bartholomew's Hospital in 1751. He shifted to St.George's Hospital in 1754 where he worked with both Cheselden and Pott, two of the most eminent surgeons in England. Throughout his years of surgical training, John continued his anatomical dissections and original research[2].

It is possible that his earliest interest was in testicular anatomy and descent[3]. In 1760, John Hunter joined the army and began to mature as a surgeon. He studied wounds and wound care that would ultimately lead to his publication in

49

1794, *A Treatise on the Blood, Inflammation, and Gun-shot Wounds*. In 1763, he retired from the army and took up residence in Golden Square to begin a private surgical practice. He was supplementing his income by teaching anatomy. His interest in unusual specimens, skill at dissection, and a keen sense of displaying his work led him to be elected to a surgeon at St. George's on 9 December 1768. He became the physician extraordinary to King George III in 1776[2].

In early 1786 he published perhaps his best known work, *Treatise on the Venereal Disease*, where he reported the natural history of gonorrhoea and syphilis by autoexperimentation[4]. Hunter had begun to inoculate his own penis with syphilis and gonorrhoea just prior to his marriage. He had to prolong his engagement until he could treat his self-induced disease[1]. Later that same year he published *Observations on Certain Parts of the Animal Economy*.

But it is Hunter's attention to the urological realm that is the focus of this investigation, and it is to his lesser known posthumous work of 1837 that we must turn, *The Works of John Hunter, F.R.S. with Notes* hereafter referred to as *The Works*[5]. This particular manuscript was completed by James F. Palmer, the senior surgeon at St. George's. It includes some of Hunter's notes and thoughts about anatomical research that was being pursued. *The Works* will form the basis of the observations regarding urological interests of Mr. Hunter coupled with biographical data.

Materials and Methods

John Hunter had a significant interest in the urinary tract and its diseases and surgical ramifications. In *The Works* Hunter demonstrat-

4
Hunter, J. *A Treatise on Venereal Disease*. Privately printed: London, 1786.

5
Hunter, J. *The Works of John Hunter*. Palmer, J. (Ed.), 4 volumes. Longman, Rees, Orme, Brown, and Breen: London, 1835.

ed his anatomical fascination with the urethra, the prostate, the bladder, upper tract involvement, and manipulations of pathologic lesions. In addition, he began to develop an interest in the undescended testicle, and hermaphrodism. He lavishly illustrates his anatomical research with outstanding drawings. The series of anatomical plates in *The Works* were prepared by several artists. This series included the now famous plate XV of the prostate. In addition, special attention was given to plates XVIII, XIX, XXV, XXVI, XXVI*, XXVII, XXVIII and XXIX which demonstrate Hunter's interest in the testicle and understanding of testicular descent. Plates XXX through XXXIII show a hermaphroditic cow[5].

Results

In Hunter's collected works, there is strong evidence that he was aware of the complexities of pathology affecting the lower urinary tract. In addition, he included the blown-out hydronephrotic ureter and kidney from one unfortunate patient. Hunter clearly demonstrated urethral stricture disease and illustrated how a surgeon can manipulate an instrument beyond an obstruction to alleviate suffering. His final series of illustrations concerned the male testicles and their descent and growth. He concluded his series with a fascinating look at a hermaphroditic cow. The best way to appreciate Hunter's fascination with genitourinary anomalies is to review his actual illustrations with his commentaries.

Plate XV is the classic illustration of the prostate utilised by several previous authors in urologic works. Hunter showed a ball-valving middle lobe that he labels "C" and called a tumour in his notes. Not mentioned were the relative thinness of this bladder and lack of

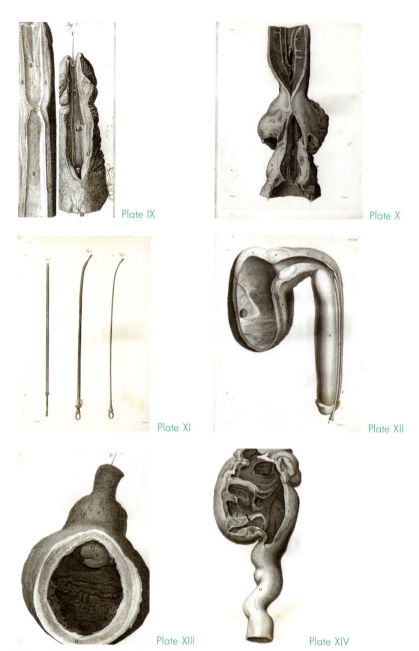
Figure 1: Series of John Hunter's lower urinary tract obstruction illustrations.

trabeculations. The prostate itself was relatively small. But Hunter drew attention to an instrument injury to the "tumour" or middle lobe[5].

The remaining series of illustrations, plates IX through XV (Fig. 1), which all have a common theme of lower urinary tract obstruction; culminated in the already mentioned, plate XV. His commentaries during this series are upon the particulars of the case, including the instruments utilised to treat the patients. Plate IX is a cutaway view of a complex urethral stricture. There is no clinical history accompanying this illustration. A close-up view of the urethral stricture is shown, and could be easily utilised in any modern treatise on stricture disease. Plate X is another stricture with attention to the urethra, both proximal and distal to the disease. The prostate was also enlarged (BB), and he demonstrated a bougie passing from the healthy towards the unhealthy portions of the urethra. A small bougie was shown lodged in a false passage. Plate XI showed the urinary instruments utilised to treat urethral diseases. One can almost sense Hunter's desire for teaching with his illustrations. He would model and practice *in vitro* prior to attempting clinical application *in vivo*. Plate XII is the first in the series with a clinical history.

The patient died of "mortification of the bladder in consequence to of a stricture and stone in the urethra." He tried to demonstrate how canulas could be utilised to deliver caustic chemicals that could have "destroyed" the stricture. Here in the bladder, an additional stone resides and the bladder was fasciculated and thickened. Plate XIII has no clinical history, but he described the pathology. An enlarged prostate with "valvular process, which has increased

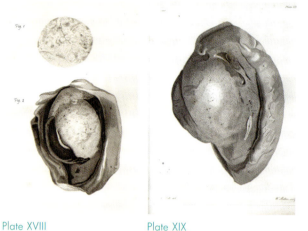

Figure 2: Initial series of testicular anatomy. This patient presented after a hydrocele drainage procedure. Hunter was instructed to try to inject the vessels with mercury to better visualise the vasculature.

Plate XVIII   Plate XIX

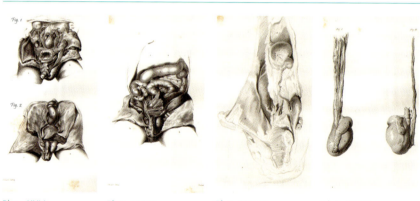

Plate XXV   Plate XXVI   Plate XXVI*   Plate XXVII

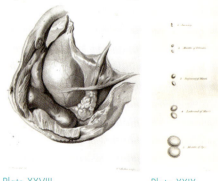

Figure 3: Hunter's series of testicular descent and growth. Human foetus are in Plates XXV and XXVI. The ram is Plate XXVI*. Human testicular blood supply injection is shown in Plate XXVII. Congenital anomalies of the vas deferens and ejaculatory apparatus is noted in plate XXVIII. Finally, Plate XXIX represents rapid testicular growth in birds (sparrows).

Plate XXVIII   Plate XXIX

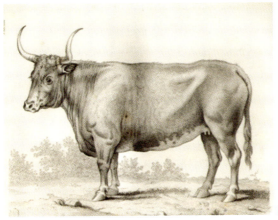
Plate XXX

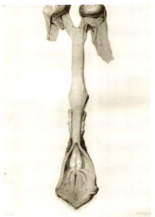
Plate XXXI

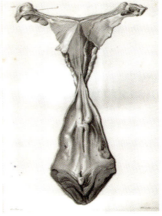
Plate XXXII

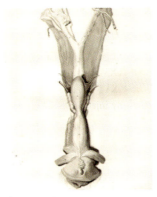

Figure 4: Hunter's final group is called Mr. Wright's free martin. He states, "It's neither like the bull nor cow."

Plate XXXIII

55

observed the development from January through April, "the beginning of the breeding season." "If we compare their size in January, with what is in April, it hardly appears possible that such wonderful change could have taken place during so short a period[5]."

This brings us to the last series of illustrations, that of the hermaphrodite. These are Plates XXX through XXXIII, which is a Mr. Wright's free martin. "It is neither like the bull nor cow." The anatomy of the hermaphrodite follows (Fig. 4)[5]. Hunter developed some theories regarding hermaphrodism and the development of gender. In his study of the freemartins he presented his notion that male and female gender might be a consequence to hermaphrodism. "Is there ever, in the genera of animals that are natural hermaphrodites, a separation of the two parts forming distinct sexes? If there is, it may account for the distinction of sexes ever having happened.[5]"

Conclusions

John Hunter's insatiable curiosity went beyond areas of surgical and anatomical research that opened new frontiers in medicine. He was voraciously interested in both anatomy and physiology. His questioning intellect prompted him to investigate everything about surgery and anatomy, not trusting in the words of others. He carried this intellectual curiosity with him into the clinical realm[6]. He has been called the reluctant surgeon by some, but he came upon this trait by both of his great surgical mentors, Cheselden and Pott. Hunter's vast experience in human cadaver dissection dwarfed any previous investigator or surgeon and by his own estimate, might have numbered in the thousands.

[6] Hunter, J. *The Case Books of John Hunter*, FRS. Allen E., Turk, J.L. and Murley R. (Eds.). Royal Society of Medicine: London, 1993.

In addition, he clinically championed *in vivo* practice by his students utilising specimens and illustrations to gain skill. He first noted the congenital hernia associated with testicular descent, and described the association of testicular anomalies with other genitourinary pathology. Finally, Hunter greatly contributed to genitourinary knowledge as well as generation. He dissected a male who died during intercourse and created a demonstration of the genitals with sperm emission. He dissected many pregnant females at various stages of gestation for his brother. He performed several Caesarean sections. Finally he developed artificial insemination of silk worms and actually helped an infertile male with hypospadias impregnate his wife utilising a warmed syringe to collect the semen and insert the fluid into the woman's vagina[7]. Hunter was also an outspoken opponent to popular medical opinions regarding the evils of masturbation and onanism, heralded by Samuel Tissot's book[1].

John Hunter should rightfully be considered the father of experimental surgery, a gifted anatomist, comparative anatomist, a physiologist, and theoretician. He also demonstrated a particular interest in genitourinary anatomy and pathology. Add to John Hunter's wide ranging surgical/anatomical interests a prescient foreshadowing of urological subspecialisation. His illustrations of both urethral pathology and synchronous utilisation of catheters and bougies is modern. He obviously attempted to utilise them in education in a fashion similar to Vesalius' use of *Tabulae Sex*.

[7] Cornelius, E.H. "John Hunter as an expert witness". *Ann Roy Coll Surg Engl.* 1978. 60:412-418.

[8] Cook, B. 'Contributions of the Hunter Brothers to our understanding of reproduction". An exhibition from the University's Library Collections. Glasgow Univ. Library, Special Collections, 1992.

Correspondence to:
Michael E. Moran
Southwest Urology
1100 N. Eldorado Pl., Tucson, AZ 34990, USA
E-mail: memoran2@juno.com

PATTISON FASCIA: THE FORGOTTEN EPONYM?

Dirk Schultheiss

Chairman History Office EAU, Department of Urology, Protestant Hospital Gießen, Germany.

Denonvilliers Fascia is a term known to all urologists. It is one of the most important surgical landmarks of the small pelvis, separating the prostate/posterior bladder wall from the anterior rectum wall. Granville Sharp Pattison described this structure in 1820 and pointed out that it absolutely must be protected during a perineal lithotomy operation. Yet this fascia is not known under his name, but under that of Denonvilliers; the man who would not describe it until 16 years later.

Introduction

Until the middle of the 19th century, the field of academic anatomical studies was, at most universities, performed in the field of surgery, which, at that point, was not academic but mainly surgically oriented. Here the so-called "barber-surgeons" functioned as demonstrators as they were the ones to dissect corpses and perform relatively rare "classical" operations on corpses. Until about 1800, this was not linked to clinical activities such as the demonstration of acute cases at the bedside. Then the anatomic knowledge could be transferred into surgical activity. This was reflected in an impressive manner in the studies of the Scottish anatomist and surgeon Granville Sharp Pattison (1791-1851) in his article about the "fascia of the prostate gland"[10]. Even the title of this work, published in America in the year 1820, is already notably clear and comprehensive: "Experimental observations on the operation of lithotomy, with the description of

[10] Pattison, G.S. "Observations on Lithotomy". *Am Med Recorder.* 1820. 3:1–24.

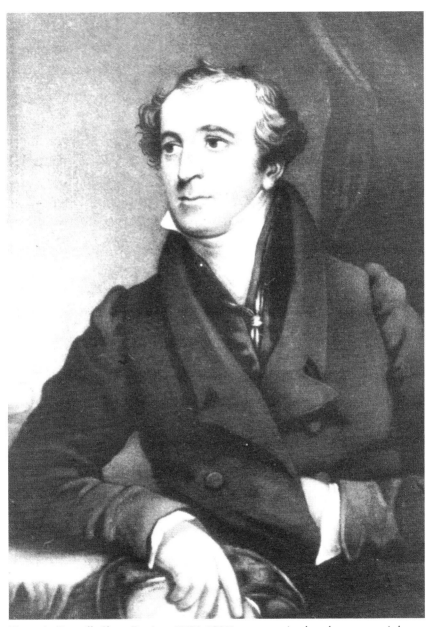

Figure 1: Granville Sharp Pattison (1791-1851): an engraving based on a portrait by Chester Harding, 1826.

a fascia of the prostate gland which appears to explain anatomically the cause of urinal infiltrations and consequent death". In it, Pattison fully described the protective function of this fascia, located between the prostate and the rectum, against infections; and, by detailing his anatomical studies, he put forward certain direct technical operative improvements for the perineal lithotomy.

Today, however, this fascia is solidly linked to the "proper name" - that of the French anatomist and surgeon Charles-Pierre Denonvilliers (1808-1872), a man who did not lecture on his anatomical treatment process until 1836, in Paris[3]. It raises questions as to why, in the continuing history of medicine, it was his name that remained in connection with such an important structure in the field of pelvic surgery. This issue is discussed in this work. The article also sheds some light on the relationship between Europe and North America in the field of medicine during the 20th century. Although the European Pattison was known as one of the leading English-speaking anatomy lecturers in Baltimore between 1820 and 1826, his writings were clearly no longer recognised some 75 years later - Hugh Hampton Young, in his writings on prostatic surgery does not mention Pattison but uses the eponym "Denonvilliers" from the European literature.

Pattison: a lively biography on two continents

Granville Sharp Pattison had a sparkling yet quarrelsome and contradictory personality. To one person he was formidable in the fields of anatomy and surgery and an academic teacher; to another he was spurned as a grave robber, an adulterer, a duellist and a chroni-

[3] Denonvilliers, C.P. "Anatomie du périnée". *Bull Soc Anat Paris.* 1836. 11:105–107.

cally quarrelsome fellow. A detailed biography about Pattison was published in 1987 by one his descendents from which the essential information contained in the following section was extracted. This carried the sub-title "anatomist and antagonist", thus summarising the ambivalent being of Pattison very aptly.

Granville Sharp Pattison was born on 23 January 1791, the son of a rich businessman and cloth producer based in Glasgow. He would later state 1793 as the year of his birth[6]. After attending the Glasgow Grammar School he studied medicine in his home town between 1806 and 1812; by 1813, in addition to his surgical activity, he already had a position as Lecturer for Anatomy at the College Street Medical School. At this time, his early career was overshadowed by legal proceedings in connection with grave robbing; although he managed to get acquitted one year later. In the years that followed he was able to gain major recognition as an anatomy lecturer; and in 1818 he was awarded the Chair for Anatomy and Surgery at the Anderson's Institution in Glasgow. Sensational was a hot dispute he had in 1816 with his superior, a surgeon at the Glasgow Royal Infirmary, in connection with two cases of inadequate patient treatment; it very nearly came to a pistol duel between the two. Between 1817 and 1819, a fellow academic - the Professor for Natural History and Chemistry Andrew Ure (1778-1858) started a suit against Pattison, whom he accused of having an affair with his wife.

As a result, Pattison readily accepted an invitation to Philadelphia in 1819; he was to conduct private anatomy lectures as a prom-

6
Miller, W.S. "Granville Sharp Pattison". *Johns Hopkins Hospital Bull.* 1919. 30: 98-104.

ised chair did not materialise. At this time Philadelphia, where in 1765 the first American medical faculty at the College of Philadelphia was established, was already a leading medical teaching institution in the United States and enjoying a good reputation. Here Pattison entangled himself in a violent and insulting argument with Nathaniel Chapman (1780-1853), who had been a Professor for the Theory and Practice of Medicine since 1808. By 1823 this led to a pistol duel with Chapman's brother-in-law, General Thomas Cadwalader (1779-1841), a scion of one of the leading families in Pennsylvania.

During this time he published his findings on the fascia of the prostate gland, and the below-listed controversy on the subject with the surgeon William Gibson. In 1820, Pattison was nominated as a Professor of Surgery in Baltimore, Maryland. Pattison was to teach in Baltimore for 6 years; many regarded him as the best living lecturer on anatomy - one who had gained considerable acclaim and fame among his students. Pattison played a decisive role in the founding of the Baltimore Infirmary, a precursor of modern hospitals. This can be seen as Pattison's pivotal contribution to the field of medicine and medical education in the United States.

In spite of this, in 1826 Pattison followed a call back to England as the Founding Professor of Anatomy at the new University of London. However the Scot Pattison was met with British rejection which culminated in a student demonstration - Pattison was dismissed in 1831.

Thus Pattison moved again to the new continent and in 1832 accepted a position of Professor of Anatomy at the Jefferson Medical College in Philadelphia. In 1841, he became one of the founders of the new Medical Department of the University of New York, where he practiced as a Professor for General Descriptive and Surgical Anatomy until his death in 1851.

Pattison married Scotswoman Mary Sharpe in New York, on 1 June 1833. It was a successful relationship - one which possibly contributed to calming Pattison's mood somewhat, encouraging him to practice his life in a less turbulent manner. He had interests besides medicine - for example, he actively supported the erection of the Grand Opera House in New

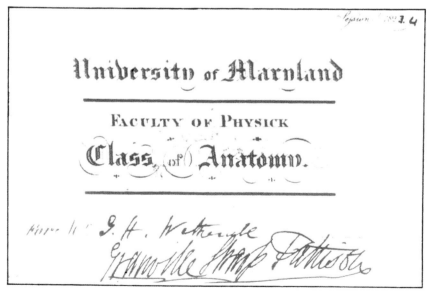

Figure 2: Entry certificate for Pattison's anatomy lecture at the University of Maryland in Baltimore 1823/249.

York. Granville Sharp Pattison died on 12th November 1851, in New York, from the results of chronic cholecystitis. His body was transferred to Scotland in the following year, and he was buried in the family grave at the Glasgow Necropolis.

Fascia of the prostrate gland: the controversial introduction

Granville Sharp Pattison announced the discovery of a new kind of fascia the moment he arrived in Philadelphia, in the summer of 1819. In the following months, he would demonstrate his findings to a number of colleagues in the fields of anatomy and surgery. Then, in January 1820, he published his findings in the American Medical Recorder (Fig. 2), a journal in which Pattison discussed "experimental observations on the operation of lithotomy, with the description of a fascia of the prostate gland which appears to explain anatomically the cause of urinal infiltrations and consequent death"[10].

The article, which delves into comprehensive detail and is 24 pages long, contains two anatomical plates, and it begins with two personal case reports from Glasgow, in which Pattison had performed a perineal lithotomy and where he even directed the autopsy following an episode in which a patient died. The opening of the abdominal cavity revealed no intraperitoneal inflammation in the small pelvis area. Only by opening the peritoneum separating the bladder from the rectum, was he able to find suppurating inflammation between the bladder wall and the seminal vesicles. Contrary to the opinions of many other authors, who stated that haemorrhage caused by perineal lithotomy was the cause of a fatal outcome, Pattison stated that these inflammations, caused by urine extravasation, were the main cause.

In this article follow accurate anatomical dissection instructions for the deep-lying fascia, stretching from between the prostate and the rectum, identified by Pattison; there is also a reference to a protective border between the perineum and the abdominal cavity. To the modern reader, there is no doubt that this is indeed the *prostato-péritonéale aponévrose* discussed by Denonvilliers 16 years later.

As the article continues, Pattison outlined how it is possible to use special surgical techniques and modified instruments to protect the fascia of the prostate and thereby prevent the above-described inflammatory urine infiltration.

Pattison finished his article by referring to earlier investigations carried out by Mr. Collies from Dublin; he emphasised that this man had outlined a different structure and did not come to the same technical surgical conclusions.

The final passage is essentially a reaction to the looming heated controversy between Pattison and William Gibson (1788-1868), Professor of Surgery at the University of Pennsylvania. Gibson had accused Pattison of plagiarism, claiming that the fascia discovered by Pattison had already been discovered in 1811 by the Irish surgeon Abraham Colles (1773-1843), who described it in the monograph *A treatise on surgical anatomy*[1]. A close examination of the article "Anatomy of the pelvis - bladder" in Colles' publication, makes it clear that he describes other anatomical structures and that

[1] Colles, A. *A treatise on surgical anatomy*. Gilbert and Hodges. Dublin, 1811, pp. 18-192.

the (named after him) "Colles Fascia" is not the structure described by Pattison.

Every argument that was put forth by either Pattison or Gibson was followed by a counter argument: this undignified and public argument was only concluded after nearly a year. The vaguely-described separation between Pattison's prostatic fascia and the Colles' fascia was adopted by other authors later on[6] and even entered in the otherwise very detailed and accurate biography[9] by F.L.M. Pattison of 1987.

How the eponym came about

In the year 1836, Charles-Pierre Denonvilliers (1808-1872) delivered a lecture to the Anatonomical Society in Paris[3] on "perineal anatomy", in which he described a layer between the seminal vesicles, the prostate and the rectum; he initially referred to this as the "prostate-peritoneal membrane layer". A year later he gave a more detailed anatomical description in the form of his dissertation; in which he introduced the term "prostate-peritoneal aponevrosis"[4]. Denonvilliers never discussed any clinical implications, and especially no operative technical details in his works[5, 7, 8].

However the Denonvilliers fascia did not become a properly established clinical and surgical term until the beginning of the 20th century - as the introduction of the radical perineal prostatectomy led to a new and intensive study of the anatomical structures of the small pelvis and especially the layers between the prostate and the rectum.

Already in 1900 Robert Proust (1873-1935; brother of author Marcel Proust) in

4
Denonvilliers, C.P. *Propositions et observations d'anatomie, de physiologie et de pathologie. Thèse de l'école de medicine.* Paris, 1837.

5
Dietrich, H. "Giovanni Domenico Santorini (1681-1737) - Charles-Pierre Denonvilliers (1808-1872): first description of urosurgically relevant structures in the small pelvis". *Eur Urol.* 1997. 32:124-127.

7
Ophoven, A., Roth, S. "Die Denonvilliers'sche Faszie". *Akt Urol.* 1996. 27: 50-51.

8
Ophoven, A., Roth, S. "The anatomy and embryological origins of the fascia of Denonvilliers: a medico-historical debate". *J Urol.* 1997. 157:3-9.

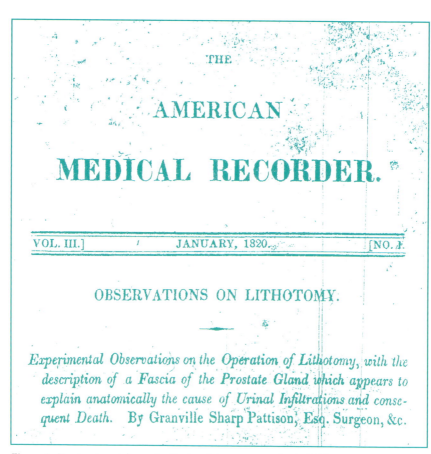

Figure 3: Pattison's article on the fascia of the prostate gland, 1820.

11
Proust, R. *De la prostatectomie périnéale totale. Thèse pour le doctorat en medicine.* Paris, 1900.

2
Cunéo, B., Veau, V. "De la signification morphologique des aponévroses périvésicales". *J Anat Physiol.* 1899. 35:235-245.

15
Pattison, F.L.M. *Granville Sharp Pattison: anatomist and antagonist, 1791-1851.* Canongate: Edinburgh, 1987.

9
Young, H.H. *A surgeon's autobiography.* Harcourt and Brace: New York, 1940.

Paris had discussed in much detail the basic principles of this new approach[11] in his doctoral publication *Total Peritoneal Prostatectomy*. In his anatomical and surgical descriptions he also discussed the "Denonvilliers' fascia". At least in the French literature this eponym must have been in use and Proust, because of regional and linguistic proximity, must have been familiar with the writings of Denonvilliers. Only a year earlier B. Cunéo and V. Veau, both prosectors in the medical faculty of Paris, had published an in-depth anatomical article on the "perivesical aponevroses" and referred to Denonvilliers[2].

In the USA, the concept of radical perineal prostatectomy was introduced by Hugh Hampton Young (1870-1945), father of American Urology, at Johns Hopkins in Baltimore, when he performed the first such operation in 1904 and was developed in the subsequent decades to a standard procedure[15]. Even Young used the eponym Denonvilliers since he obviously was not familiar with Pattison's work. This is remarkable since even in 1902, Sir William Osler (1849-1919), who was the first Professor of Medicine at the John Hopkins University in Baltimore, from 1888 to 1905, drew attention to the extraordinary biography of Granville Sharp Pattison[9]. In 1918, William Snow Miller delivered a lecture on the life of Pattison to the Johns Hopkins Hospital Historical Club and published it in detail a year later in the Johns Hopkins Hospital Bulletin[6].

Hugh Hampton Young was obviously intensively occupied with the anatomy of the Denonvilliers fascia - he would later even initiate a study of the embryological origin of this structure. This work was begun by Miley

B. Weston at the John Hopkins Hospital in Baltimore and completed at the University of California in San Francisco. It was published in the *Journal of Urology* in 1922[14]. It also contains an historical outline, though Pattison was not mentioned at all.

It was not until 1969 that the significance of Pattison's work would be formally voiced and emphasised, in a medical history article on the advances in relation to lithotomic surgery; it claimed that Denonvilliers had described the same anatomical structure more than a decade later while totally neglecting a discussion of any clinical implications. The authors of this article note, with very cautious surprise, that anatomists and surgeons, over the course of time, showed preference for the name Denonvilliers rather than that of the original author, Pattison[13]. But this reference has not been recognized up to this day - even the most recent works on the history of medicine relevant to the Denonvilliers fascia bear no reference to the earlier and more significant work of Pattison[5, 7, 8].

Epilogue

In his publication from the year 1820, Granville Sharp Pattison was the first to clearly describe the clinical and surgical importance of the dorsal prostatic fascia, and recognise the intra-operative injury of this as the cause of a lethal urinary extravasation towards the rectum. The protection of this fascia between posterior surfaces of the prostate and rectum during the then-standard operation of the perineal lithotomy was a very clear postulate and may have been a tremendous step forward on the road to avoidance of fatal post-operative wound

[14] Wesson, M.B. "The development and surgical importance of the rectourethralis muscle and Denonvilliers' fascia". *J Urol*. 1922. 8:339-359.

[13] Wangensteen, O.H., Wangensteen, S.D., Wiita, J. "Lithotomy and lithotomists: progress in wound management from Franco to Lister". *Surgery*. 1969. 66:929–952.

infections. It remains difficult to understand why this so important anatomical structure for urological surgeons was ascribed to and given the name of Denonvilliers in the later history of medicine. Charles-Pierre Denonvilliers published his description only in 1836 and did not see any surgical or clinical relevance.

Research in the development of prostatic surgery beginning with the 20th century showed a new focal point. Important anatomical contributions of these days initially came from Europe; the authors were probably more familiar with the work of Denonvilliers than that of Pattison. It remains unclear why even the later pioneers of urology in Baltimore, the most effective workplace of Pattison between 1820 and 1826, did not mention his name as an eponym whether during the development of the first radical perineal prostatectomy (Hugh H. Young, 1904) as well as the nerve-sparing retropubic prostatectomy (Patrick C. Walsh, 1982)[12].

[12] Walsh P. "Anatomic radical prostatectomy: evolution of the surgical technique". *J Urol.* 1998. 160: 2418-2424.

Correspondence to:
Dirk Schultheiss
Urology Office
Friedrichstr. 21, 35392 Gießen
Email: dirk.schultheiss@urologie-giessen.de

DO UNTO YOURSELF AS YOU WOULD DO TO OTHERS - SELF EXPERIMENTATION IN UROLOGY

Johanna Thomas, Omer Karim, Hanif Motiwala and Amrith Raj Rao

Department of Urology, Wexham Park Hospital, Berkshire, UK.

Well in that case there's another way to prove it's not dangerous, I'll experiment on myself.
Werner Forssmann, 1929

Progress in medicine is often made due to unexpected research by scientists experimenting on themselves. Novel theories are met with disbelief when presented, and as a consequence scientists can be forced to try out their hypotheses using themselves as a subject. Their strong belief in their own ideas has resulted in many of the modern advances in medicine witnessed in the 20th century. We explored the scientific literature to see if such experimentation had made an impact on progress in urology.

John Hunter (1728 - 1793)

John Hunter is known as the father of modern surgery. In his era he was unique in providing an experimental basis to surgical practice.

In the middle of the 18th century venereal disease and complaints comprised a large proportion of John Hunter's work. Sexually transmitted infections such as gonorrhoea and syphilis were rampant in Georgian London. One publication offering careers advice for young men in 1747 remarked that three out of four surgeons in London were reliant for their income in treating venereal infections[1].

1
Moore, W. *The Knife Man.* 2005.

Hunter was aware that venereal diseases were transmitted by sexual contact, but his understanding ended there. Along with most practitioners of his day Hunter believed that gonorrhoea and its more serious "cousin" syphilis, were simply different forms of the same disease. Classic symptoms of gonorrhoea (or "the Clap" as it was known) were regarded as the local manifestation of this venereal infection, affecting only the genitals. Symptoms of syphilis ('the Pox') were observed in patients once the "poison" had circulated around the body, or in Hunter's terms, had become "constitutional". Hunter felt that no two diseases could occupy one body at the same time.

On a Friday in May 1767, John Hunter embarked on an unusual experiment. Hunter set out to prove his theory, that gonorrhoea and syphilis were indeed different manifestations of the same disease. He resolved to inoculate a person with gonorrhoea and monitor the progress of the disease for signs of syphilis. If, as he expected, the signs of gonorrhoea were followed by symptoms of syphilis then he could prove that the two were one disease, but if no signs of syphilis emerged, gonorrhoea was a separate disease[1,2].

Hunter needed a compliant and willing volunteer and also someone who he could be sure had previously been clear of venereal infection. This person would also need to be willing to undergo regular examination and treatment; someone he could observe on an almost daily basis over the long course of his trial. The obvious subject was himself, although this is still the subject of some contention[5].

[2] Herman, J.R. "Syphilis and Gonorrhoea are one disease, John Hunter". *Int J Derm.* 1978. 17:252-255.

[5] Qvist, G. "Hunterian Oration 1979". *Annals of the Royal College of Surgeons of England.* 1979. 61.

Hunter took a scalpel and dipped the blade into a festering venereal sore of an infected man's penis. He then jabbed the blade first into the end and then into the foreskin of the penis. He recorded the entire process. He ensured that the identity of the subject was obscured throughout using neither the first nor the third person in his documentation[4].

> Two punctures were made on the penis with a lancet dipped in venereal matter from a gonorrhoea; one puncture was on the glans, the other on the prepuce. This was on a Friday; on the Sunday following there was a teasing and itching in those parts, which lasted till the Tuesday following[1,2].
>
> Upon the Tuesday morning the parts of the prepuce where the puncture had been made were redder, thickened and had formed a speck; by the Tuesday following the speck had increased and discharged some matter, and there seemed to be a little pouting of the lips of the urethra, also a sensation in it in making water, so that a discharge was expected from it.

Hunter went on to document that within ten days, an ulcer or chancre appeared on the foreskin and soon other signs of syphilis emerged. Two months later " a little sharp pricking pain was felt in one of the tonsils". On examination this proved to be an ulcer, a common occurrence in the primary stage of syphilis. Seven months after the start of the experiment 'copper-coloured blotches' broke out on the skin, clearly indicating that syphilis had entered its secondary stage.

For Hunter the experiment was a success and proved his hypothesis. Hunter published his findings in his treatise on venereal disease in 1786. However, the patient whom he chose with signs of gonorrhoea to obtain the venereal matter from was obviously also infected with *Treponema palidum*. The results of this fated trial would set back medical progress in terms of the understanding of sexually transmitted infections by half a century. It was not until 1838 when the French-based physician Phillip Ricord established that the two diseases were indeed separate, after conducting his own series of inoculation experiments on a remarkable unwitting 2500 patients[2].

Hunter would never reveal the name of the guinea pig - the identity of the subject would be a cause of debate for the next two centuries[5]. The idea that Hunter would have willingly inflicted on himself such a vile disease as syphilis was inconceivable to many of his later devotees. However, according to the notes of his pupils, he is recorded having talked in the first person about this experiment. By the time Hunter's collected works appeared in 1835, the surgeon who edited the venereal disease treatise, George Babbington would state that Hunter performed the experiment on himself [1,3].

3
Dempster, W. "Towards a new understanding of John Hunter". *Lancet*. 1978. 316-318.

Wilhelm Roentgen (1845-1923)

Wilhelm Roentgen was a German physicist who earned the first Nobel Prize for Physics for his discovery of X-rays. On 8 November 1895 he produced and detected electromagnetic radiation in a wavelength that we know today as X-rays.

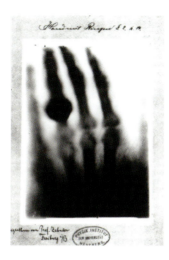

Figure 1: X-ray of Wilhelm Roentgen's wife's hand. On seeing this she said: "Now I have seen my death."

He discovered X-rays whilst investigating the external effects from various types of vacuum tube equipment when an electrical discharge is passed through them. One of the vacuum tubes had a thin aluminum window added to the end of the tube to allow cathode rays to exit the tube. A cardboard covering had been added to protect the cathode rays. Roentgen observed that the invisible cathode rays exiting from the tube caused a fluorescent effect on a small cardboard screen painted with barium platinocyanide when working in a dark room. During subsequent experiments he found that objects of different thickness interposed in the path of the X-rays showed variable transparency to them when recorded on a photographic plate. He X-rayed his own hand and his wife's hand, to show that bones could be identified from the images[6] (Fig. 1).

X-rays today are an indispensable part of the investigation and management of urological disease. There is no record that Roentgen suffered from the ill effects of the radiation he was exposed to during these experiments.

[6] Glaser, O. *Wilhelm Roentgen and the early history of the Roentgen rays.* 1993.

Friedrich Meyer-Betz

Photodynamic therapy is a treatment option for superficial bladder tumours. The therapy is a potentially selective approach in which in-situ photosensitisation by a non-toxic drug, locally activated by light, generates cytotoxic reactive oxygen species, causing cell death.

The concept was first identified in 1879 when medical student Oscar Raab, working in the pharmacology lab of Professor Von Tappeiner, examined effects of dyestuffs on paramecia (unicellular organisms). He observed that when using a low concentration of acridine as the photosensitizer, the paramecia were killed in the presence of daylight, but survived in the darkness. Further research within this field by Hans Fielder showed that haematoporphyrin

Figure 2: Meyer- Betz three days after photosensitisation, note how the right side of his face is more oedematous and it was this part that was more exposed to the sunlight.

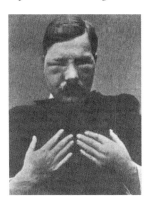
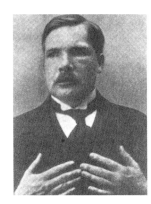

Figure 3: Meyer-Betz five days after photo-sensitisation.

had a strong photodynamic effect when injected subcutaneously into the mouse.

Friedrich Meyer-Betz was an Austrian physician and had been a co-worker of Hans Fischer. Working in the medical clinic at Konigsberg he carried out a remarkable experiment on himself.

Between 05:45 and 06:15 on 14 October 1912 he injected himself intravenously with 200mg of haematoporphyrin. The next day was overcast and nothing spectacular occurred. The following day on 16 October it was a sunny day and a photosensitised reaction set in. Meyer-Betz described it as a prickling and burning sensation, with those regions of his body which had been exposed to sunlight developing erythema and oedema. Meyer-Betz had exposed the right side of his face more than the left side. This shows clearly in the photo taken on 17 October. By 19 October the oedema had lessened, but the photosensitivity remained for several weeks until the haematoporphyrin had been metabolised[7] (Figs. 2, 3).

Werner Forssmann (1904-1979)

Werner Forssmann was the pioneer of cardiac catheterisation in man. Dissatisfied with the inaccuracy and uncertainty of heart diagnosis, Forssmann dreamt of efficient heart surgery that required a route of access to the great vessels. Until the late 1920s, standard methods of cardiac diagnosis were percussion, auscultation, X-ray and ECG. As a student, Forssmann was fascinated by experiments on animal physiology performed by Claude Bernard and his contemporaries. They used horses as subjects and had introduced a catheter into both the right and left ventricles using a retrograde approach from

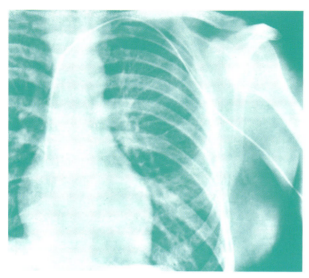

Figure 3: X-ray taken by Forssmann showing the tip of the ureteral catheter lying within the right ventricle.

the jugular vein and carotid artery [8]. Forssmann was convinced that this experimental arrangement could also be used on man without any danger. In 1929 at the age of 25, while doing his surgical training at Eberswalde, a small town near Berlin, he introduced a ureteral catheter into his own right arm and walked up a flight of stairs to the X-ray department. He took an X-ray, which showed the tip of the catheter at the head of the humerus. He then advanced the catheter further up to 65cm so that the catheter tip was seen passing into the right ventricle[9,10] (Fig. 4). His original article, entitled "Probing the right ventricle of the heart", was published on 5 November 1929 in *Klinische Wochenschrift*.

Forssmann had two objects in mind. Firstly to use this technique in emergencies to

[8] Baim, D., Grossman, W. *Grossman's cardiac catheterisation, angiography and intervention.* 2005.

[9] Forssmann, W. *Experiments on myself: Memoirs of a surgeon in Germany.* 1974.

[10] Corbin N, Thompson I, Urology and the Nobel Prize, *Urologic Oncology: Seminars and Original Investigations.* 2003. 21: 83-85

administer drugs directly into the heart, and secondly "to study the heart and for diagnosis". Altogether he catheterised his own heart nine times without any side effects. He also injected contrast material, Uroselectan, in 1931 in an attempt to produce an angiocardiogram[9]. By 1932 pulmonary angiography using a catheter in the right atrium had been done in Lisbon, Paris, and Buenos Aires. He finally stopped using himself as a subject when attempting contrast radiography of the aorta through his back. He attempted this three times, and each time he experienced a sharp stabbing pain. He decided, along with pressure from his wife, that he should no longer continue with self-experimentation[9,12].

[12] Fontenot, C. ,O'Leary, J. "Dr. Werner Forssmann's Self-Experimentation". *American Surgeon*. 1996. 62; 6:514-515

Following the publication of his article he attempted to pursue a career in academic medicine. However, he faced bitter opposition and never succeeded in establishing himself in this field. Lectures he gave on his own experiments were met with shocked murmuring, stamping and laughter[9]. Forssmann went on to the Rudolf Virchow Hospital in Berlin for specialist training in another catheter related career in urology under Dr. Karl Heusch[8]. He was appointed Chief of the Surgical Clinic of the City Hospital at Dresden-Friedrichstadt and at the Robert Koch Hospital, Berlin. Following the outbreak of World War II he served as a Sanitary Officer, reaching the rank of Surgeon-Major. He was made a prisoner of war in 1945, but escaped and found his family living in the Schwarzwald[9,10].

His pioneering work was finally recognised in 1956 when he was awarded the Nobel Prize for physiology and Medicine, along with to make it possible to exhibit the results. He stepped around the podium, and pulled his loose pants tight up around his genitalia in an attempt to demonstrate his erection.

At this point, I, and I believe everyone else in the room, was agog. I could scarcely believe what was occurring on stage. But Professor Brindley was not satisfied. He looked down sceptically at his pants and shook his head with dismay. "Unfortunately, this doesn't display the results clearly enough". He then summarily dropped his trousers and shorts, revealing a long, thin, clearly erect penis. There was not a sound in the room. Everyone had stopped breathing.

But the mere public showing of his erection from the podium was not sufficient. He paused, and seemed to ponder his next move. The sense of drama in the room was palpable. He then said, with gravity, "I'd like to give some of the audience the opportunity to confirm the degree of tumescence". With his pants at his knees, he waddled down the stairs, approaching (to their horror) the urologists and their partners in the front row. As he approached them, erection waggling before him, four or five of the women in the front rows threw their arms up in the air, seemingly in unison, and screamed loudly. The scientific merits of the presentation had been overwhelmed, for them, by the novel and unusual mode of demonstrating the results.

The screams seemed to shock Professor Brindley, who rapidly pulled up his trousers, returned to the podium, and terminated the lecture. The crowd dispersed in a state of flabbergasted disarray. I imagine that the urologists who attended with their partners had a lot of explaining to do. The rest is history. Prof Brindley's single-author paper reporting these results was published about 6 months later[14].

Conclusion

We hope to have demonstrated how self-experimentation has had a profound effect on a variety of areas within the urological field. These courageous scientists, some after having suffered side effects from their experiments, have paved the way for the continuing advancement of medical science. We have shown that self-experimentation is not an old phenomenon and will probably continue to be used as a research tool in the future.

Correspondence to:
Johanna Thomas
58A Parfrey St, London, W6 9EN, UK
E-mail: johanna_thomas31@yahoo.co.uk

---

14 Klotz, L. "How (not) to communicate new scientific information: a memoir of the famous Brindley lecture". *BJU Int.* 2005. 96(7):956-957.

HISTORY OF THE TERM PROSTATE*

Franz Josef Marx and Axel Karenberg

Institute for the History of Medicine and Medical Ethics, University of Cologne, Cologne, Germany.

*Marx, F.J., Karenberg, A. "History of the Term Prostate". *The Prostate*. 2008. 69, 2:208-213. @ 2010 Wiley-Liss, Inc. Reprinted with permission.

[1] Douglas, L.L. "Urologic terminology and misnomers". *Urology*. 1983. 22:98.

"We, however… are convinced that the chief merit of language is clearness; accordingly we employ those terms which the bulk of people are accustomed to use". With this declaration the ancient physician Galen (129 - ca. 210 A.D.) delineated two essential aspects of any professional terminology: unambiguity and comprehensibility. These ideals have lost nothing of their validity and they characterise not only medical terminology in general, but urologic nomenclature in particular[1].

The history of many technical terms is, however, one of confusion. For example, some expressions urologists use today had completely different meanings in the past. Conversely, physical structures and symptoms with which we are familiar today often bore completely different labels in the past. However historical development did not always lead to greater precision. This hypothesis will be tested in this essay using the example of the anatomical designation "prostate".

Etymology

The origin of the name of an organ which currently stands at the centre of urological practice reaches back to ancient Greece. The original noun *prostatēs* can be parsed into three parts: the prefix *pro-* (=before), the stem *sta* (=stand), and the suffix *-tēs* (which forms agent nouns). The male substantive *prostatēs* literally means "someone who stands before someone or something", that is "president" or "principal".

89

Contemporary parlance and the literature of the 6th to the 4th century B.C. provide various usages[2]. The historian Herodotus used the word to distinguish the "leader" or "chief" of an army while Plato did so to characterise the "president" of a state. The tragedian Aeschylus used the word to characterise the "guardian" of a gate and his contemporary Sophocles did the same with reference to the "protector" of a city. The Greek verb *proístanai* means "to stand before", "to put in front" or "to stand in public". This semantic variant gave rise to the Latin verb *prostate* whose modern-day derivatives include prostitute and prostitution. The word prostatēs or its variants make no appearance in any kind of medical context, however.

Part and parcel of this story is the similarly sounding Greek word *parastatēs*. The prefix para means "next to", thus literally *parastatēs* means "someone who stands next to someone or something" or "companion". Yet in contrast to *prostatēs*, *parastatēs* was used in ancient times to indicate a part of the male reproductive system - in the plural with varying meanings and occasionally supplemented with an epithet. A few authors understood this to be the testicles or epididymides, others the spermatic ducts. They all shared the opinion that these body parts played an important "helping" role in procreation and deserved to be designated by an easily understandable metaphoric expression.

Early anatomical investigations

Surprising to modern urologists is another fact: independent of the terminological puzzle, no medical text from the ancient, Byzantine or Islamic period even mentions the unpaired prostate organ[3]. This historical silence can be

[2] Liddell, H.G., Scott, R. A Greek-English Lexikon. Clarendon: Oxford, 1991, pp.1325, 1526-1527.

[3] Barcia Goyanes, J.J. *Onomatologia anatomica nova: Historia del lenguaje anatómico*. Vol. VII. Secretariado de Publicaciones: Valencia, 1985, p. 24.

explained by the research practices of the day. Until the 14th century anatomical dissection - when possible at all - was carried out almost exclusively on animals. Yet anatomical differences between species are quite considerable. In dogs, cats, cattle and horses, for example, the glandular part of the prostate is more or less clearly divided into two lobes while in sheep and goats it is missing altogether. In contrast to herbivores, carnivores do not have seminal vesicles[4]. Zoological research thus did not help to clarify this issue very much.

For a limited time dissection of human corpses was possible in Alexandria, the scientific centre of Hellenism, around 300 B.C. Many of the discoveries made there are linked with the physician Herophilus who is therefore known as "the first anatomist". In fact the Alexandrian scholar described and named numerous parts of the male sexual organs and possibly came very close to identifying the human prostate. This conjecture is based on one of Galen's texts which summarised ancient anatomy and was of singular importance for the later denomination of the organ[5]:

> The humour produced in those glandular bodies [i.e., the seminal vesicles in current terminology] is poured into the urinary passage in the male along with the semen and its uses are to excite to the sexual act, to make coitus pleasurable, and to moisten the urinary passageway... This is the reason, I suppose, why they do not hesitate to call the passageways arising from these bodies spermatic vessels and indeed Herophilus was the first to call them "glandular

---

4

Bush, R.B., Bush, I.M. "Early developments in the history of prostatic disorders". In: Tannenbaum, M. (ed.). *Urologic pathology: The prostate*. Lea & Felbinger: Philadelphia, 1977, pp. 7-22.

5

Galen, C. *On the usefulness of the parts of the body*. Translation. Vol. II. Cornell University Press: Ithaca, 1968, p. 644.

assistants" (*parastatai adenoeides*) since he had called those that grow out from the testes "varicose assistants" (*parastatai kirsoeides*) [i.e., the ampullae of the vasa deferentia].

The strongest argument against accepting that by "glandular assistants" Herophilus meant the prostate is the fact that he used the plural form of the Greek words for both the seminal vesicles as well as for the seminal ducts - a clear indication of bilateral organs[6]. In the tradition of the Alexandrian anatomists, in 200 A.D. Galen, who also wrote in Greek, named the seminal vesicles "glandular bodies" or "semen-containing assistants"; he did not definitively identify the prostate[7]. Thus at the end of the ancient period an anatomical and terminological separation of the paired seminal vesicles and the seminal ducts had been achieved. Further advancement was only possible in that stage of the history of urology which once again permitted human autopsies for research purposes.

[6] von Staden, H. *Herophilus: The art of medicine in early Alexandria*. University Press: Cambridge, 1989, p 167.

[7] Musitelli, O., Ogliari, F. *La prostata nella storia della medicina*. Selecta medica: Pavia, 2006.

Renaissance anatomy and terminology

With respect to our subject, the Latin anatomical literature of the 16th century can be divided into three parts: the pre-Vesalian phase, characterised by mere repetition of ancient knowledge and therewith the passing on of Herophilean-Galenic terminology; the visualisation and description of the organs by Vesalius in 1538 and 1543; and the post-Vesalian period during which linguistic usage varied and the function of the organ was subject of speculation.

The difficulty of identifying the prostate in earlier human dissections is made clear by Leonardo da Vinci's anatomical studies[8]. His representations of the male genital tract, based on autopsies he conducted himself, are distinguished by an accurate and artistic reproduction of the seminal ducts and the seminal vesicles. However the prostate is not to be found in any of his drawings-perhaps because the ancient medical texts he consulted made no mention of this organ. Leonardo's drawings strongly support the idea that all of early modern anatomy was characterised by theory-driven perception. Jacopo Berengario da Carpi, professor of surgery in Pavia and Bologna and one of the most important pre-Vesalian anatomists, also mentioned only the seminal vesicles in 1520 and wrote [9]: "Galen, following Eracleus (=Herophilus), calls them *parastata adeniformia* because adenous flesh surrounds them".

The first to mention the prostate was the Venetian physician Niccolò Massa who did so in passing in his 1536 *Introductory Book of Anatomy*: "…you will find a glandular flesh upon which rests the neck of the bladder and the extremities of the aforementioned [seminal] vessels… Through these carunculae also pass the seminal vessels…" [10]

Yet it was the principal reformer of anatomy, Andreas Vesalius who drew and exactly described the prostate gland. It is first depicted in his work from 1538[11]. Five years later he described the vasa deferentia and the prostate, although not the seminal vesicles, as definitively separate organs. The prostate is localised between the bladder and the ring-shaped sphincter (Fig. 1) and is labelled in the legend and accompanying text with the unspecific designations "glandulous body" (*corpus glandulosum*)

[8] Da Vinci, L. *On the human body*. Translation. Greenwich House: New York, 1982. pp. 440-441, 444-445.

[9] Berengario daCarpi, J. *A short introduction to anatomy*. Translation. University Press: Chicago, 1959, p. 69.

[10] Massa, N. "Liber introductorius". Translation. In: Lind, L.R. (ed.). *Studies in pre-Vesalian anatomy*. American Philosophical Society: Philadelphia, 1975, pp. 199, 201.

[11] Vesalius, A. "Tabulae anatomicae". In: Saunders, J.B., O'Malley, C.D. (ed.). *The illustrations from the works of Andreas Vesalius*: Dover: New York, 1950, pp. 236–237.

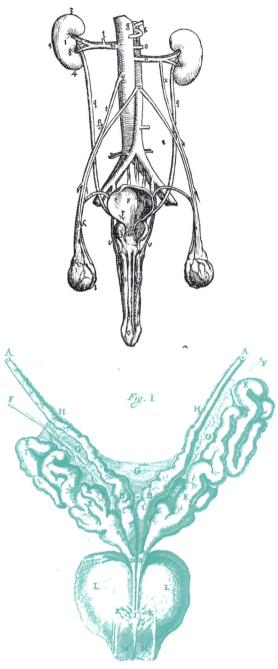

Figure 1: Anterior view of the male genitalia. Vesalius A. *Fabrica*, book V;1543. Figure XXIII, p. 374.

Figure 2: Posterior view of prostate and seminal vesicles. De Graaf, R. *Tractatus*; 1678. Table VI, figure I.

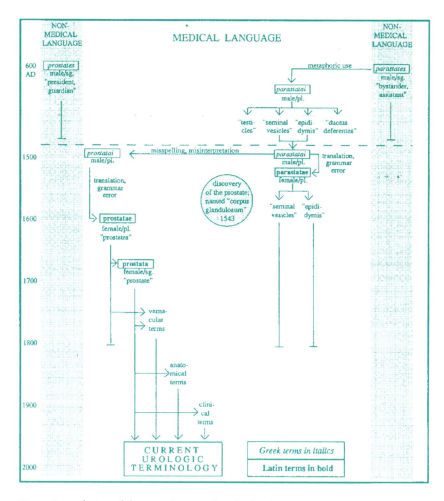

Figure 3: Evolution of the term "prostate" and related terms.

and "glandulous bystander". Thereby Vesalius singularised the Galenic term "glandular bodies" and transferred the traditional term from the well-known seminal vesicles to the newly discovered prostate[12]: "The glandulous body into which the vessels that bring down semen insert after they have come together… is located at the bottom of the bladder and its neck. It is a single body, often larger than the testes. It is not exactly round but has a depression at the front and back; at the sides it is perfectly spherical. Through the middle of it runs the vesical canal…"

[12] Vesalius, A. "On the fabric of the human body". Book V: *The organs of nutrition and generation*. Translation. Norman: Novato, 2007, pp. 155–156.

Scholars of the post-Vesalian period accepted the discovery of the organ, although they were not in agreement as to whether it was a paired or unpaired organ. With respect to its function, four different assumptions predominated. A first group of authors thought the prostate refined the semen flowing from the testicles. A second group argued that it separated a pungent whey-like fluid from the blood to arouse greater pleasure during the sexual act. A third Group maintained that it produced a fluid for moistening and protecting the urethra; and a fourth defended the notion that semen is generated in the prostate.

17th and 18th century nomenclature

In the year 1600 the French anatomist André du Laurens introduced an epochal terminological reform in that he first called the chestnut-sized formation beneath the bladder *prostatae*. Until that point it had no such Latin designation in either the ancient or the medieval periods. Although the drawing in du Laurens' textbook (virtually a copy of one of Vesalius' illustrations) showed a single, oval organ, the

[13] Du Laurens, A. *Historia anatomica*. Becker: Francoforti, 1600, pp. 194–195, 262.

corresponding text reads as follows[13]: "There [i.e., at the neck of the bladder] two very white, gland-like bodies appear, which collect and conserve the semen. Anatomists call them *prostatae*". The final sentence suggests that du Laurens was not presenting a word of his own creation, but documenting colloquial usage among scholars. However the debut of the term in professional nomenclature was accompanied by three capital errors.

1. *Historical error*: Du Laurens proceeded from the incorrect assumption that Herophilus had already discovered the organ and designated it as *prostatai adenoeides* (glandular bodies). This historical misunderstanding is partly explicable by the fact that in some late medieval codices and in editions of Galen's *On the usefulness of the parts of the body* published after 1500 the Greek word *parastatai* was incorrectly indicated by *prostatai*.

2. *Grammatical error*: Du Laurens and his contemporaries incorrectly understood the Greek word *prostatai* to be feminine which led them to translate it incorrectly into Latin as *prostatae*. Its correct Latin form would have been *prostatores* in the plural and prostator in the singular.

3. *Morphological error*: Du Laurens erroneously understood the prostate gland to be a pair of organs. The structure of the human prostate with two prominent lateral lobes may have contributed to this misperception.

In subsequent decades these errors in du Laurens' textbook were perpetuated. The most influential example is the work of the Danish anatomist Caspar Bartholin the Elder. Like his predecessors, in 1611 he characterised the *prostatae* as a spongy, paired organ that was connected to the urethra by pores and whose secretion protected the urethra. Remarkably Bartholin detected - as did Massa - the joint outlet of the seminal vesicles and seminal ducts. He was one of the first to present a (albeit partially incorrect) derivation of the term: "The *prostatae*, however, are glands, which are called by the Greeks in this manner because they are standing in front"[14].

In the anatomical literature of the 17th and 18th centuries the plural prostatae dominated. This form can be found in a well-known treatise by the Dutch anatomist Reinier De Graaf who, however, betrayed his meagre knowledge of Greek[15]: "*The prostatae*, so-called by the ancients as though they were bystanders [i.e., *parastatae*], are simply one spongy body stuffed with various tiny glands. "Nevertheless it was here that for the first time the organ was portrayed together with seminal vesicles and seminal ducts in a separate drawing (Fig. 2) which hardly differs from contemporary representations. *Prostatae* appeared likewise in the much read work by the Flemish anatomist Philipp Verheyen[16]; his account of the organ's shape, size, glands and its relation to the ejaculatory ducts was quite accurate. In 1732 Jacques Winslow, member of the Royal Academy of Science in Paris, also proceeded from the idea that the *prostate* was a double organ. Yet in 1804 the English anatomist and surgeon John Abernethy still spoke of two prostatae.

14
Bartholin, C. *Institutiones anatomiques*. Henault: Paris, 1647, p. 161.

15
De Graaf, R. "*Tractatus de virorum organis generationi inservientibus*". In: Opera omnia. Lugduni Batavorum: Hugentan, 1678, pp. 34-35.

16
Verheyen, P. *Corporis humani anatomia*. Lipsiae: Fritsch, 1705, plates IX and X, pp. 168–169.

In contrast, the singular *prostata* is only sporadically found. In 1652 the English surgeon Nathaniel Highmore, who was a friend of William Harvey, was one of the first to use this variant[17]: "...these (seminal) Atomes are separated by the testicles, a glandulous body; next, they are conveighed [sic] to the Prostata, a glandule too". The turning point in medical linguistic usage came in 1792 with a brief notation in a new edition of a textbook by the English anatomist and surgeon William Cheselden (1688-1752)[18]: "Prostatae are two glands, or rather one, about the size of a nutmeg". With refined research methods of normal and pathological anatomy as well as knowledge from surgical practice, the morphological unity of the organ could be proven around 1800[19]. From this point on the singular *prostata* began its victory march within urologic nomenclature.

The aftermath: vernacular and clinical terms

Transformation of the Greco-Latin term into modern languages had already taken place a few decades earlier. In 1711 prostate glandules was used in English[20] which by 1752 had been supplemented with prostate gland[21]. A key role played the monograph *Practical observations on the treatment of the diseases of the prostate gland* (1811) by the London-based surgeon Sir Everard Home. Home's book was largely based on unpublished manuscripts of his brother-in-law John Hunter, a famous British anatomist and surgeon. In the 19th century numerous anatomical details were recognised and named including Apex prostatae, Basis prostatae, Lobus medius, Facies vesicalis, Facies pubica and Facies rectalis. The median lobe, particularly relevant in prostatic hypertrophy, received a large number of varied designations, for example, Home's lobe, Isthmus

17
Highmore, N. *The history of generation*. Martin: London, 1651, p. 109.

18
Cheselden, W. *The anatomy of the human body*. 13th edition. Dodsley: London.

19
Murphy, L.J.T. *The history of urology*. Thomas: Springfield, 1972, pp. 379-380.

20
Marten, J. *Treatise of all the degrees and symptoms of the venereal disease*. 7th edition. Crouch: London, 1711, p. 394.

21
Smellie, W. *A treatise on the theory and practice of midwifery*. Wilson: London, 1752.

prostatae, Lobus pathologicus, Lobus inferior or *portion médiane*. Finally, in the 20th century came an abundance of clinically derived terms ranging from prostatism to prostate-specific antigen.

Conclusions

This brief survey has documented how confusing the history of the prostate and its designations have been. This history has been played out in dissection rooms and scriptoria. It has involved paired and unpaired organs, Greek and Latin, singular and plural, and male and female substantives. It has also involved fragile and inconstant relations between denominating words and significant subjects (Fig. 3):

1. The meaning of the original form *prostatēs* explains its later metaphoric use in anatomic and urologic terminology. However its first use within a medical context took place more than 2000 years after its coinage.
2. The discovery of the organ by Renaissance anatomists was not linked to a name from which the current appellation is derived.
3. The specification of the word *prostatae* by André du Laurens in 1600 was based on serious historical, linguistic and anatomical misperceptions. This neologism nevertheless prevailed for a long time.
4. With the clarification of the organ structure the Latin designation *prostata* and its English equivalent *prostate* first came into use. From this point on the increasingly specialised terminology represented a dependent variable of anatomical and clinical research.

What this overview has demonstrated via the history of the word prostate is also true of many other technical terms in urology. This expression from current nomenclature is an outstanding example of successful research into the historical layers of urology and its language. Simultaneously the dynamics of medical and terminological development imply that we can expect new words to enrich urology in the future. As Shakespeare observed: "What's past is prologue".

Acknowledgements

David D. Lee assisted with manuscript preparation.

Correspondence to:
Axel Karenberg
Institute for the History of Medicine and Medical Ethics
University of Cologne
Joseph-Stelzmann-Strasse 20
D-50931 Cologne, Germany
E-mail: ajg02@uni-koeln.de

ANDREAS VESALIUS AND SEMINAL ERRORS

Michael E. Moran

Southwest Urology, Tucson, USA

An overview

Andreas Vesalius is credited as the founder of modern medical anatomy, reawakening critical thinking and investigation with the publication from the press of Johannes Oporinus in Basel of *De humani corporis fabrica libri septum* and his Epitome in 1543.

As amazing and truly revolutionary as these textbooks are, Vesalius failed in several areas, particularly his imbedded prejudices that still linger from his understanding of classic Greek and Roman work that predates his own sentinel investigations.

Reading the *Fabrica and Epitome* a modern physician can readily appreciate the enormous undertaking of this work. This particular investigation is concerned with Vesalius' *Epitome* chapter VI "Concerning the Organs Which Minister To the Propagation of the Species" and the *Fabrica* Plates 58 & 59 regarding the urinary tract. This represents a review of his statements and anatomical descriptions of the genitourinary system.

In *Fabrica* Vesalius depicts the kidneys lying *in situ* within the retroperitoneum. Close-up bivalved canine kidneys, clearly labelled, represent his hypothesis that the kidneys contained no sieves, the current popular hypothesis of Gabriele de Zerbis.

He states that the canine kidney was chosen in this representation because it was less fatty than the human. He clearly demonstrates no sieve system yet he offers no alternative. His plate 59 demonstrates the lower urinary tract with genital structures including the prostate and the ampullae of the vas deferens all clearly recognisable. A close-up of the testicle shows an anatomically correct epididymis.

Vesalius demonstrates an uncanny ability to observe and demonstrate anatomy. Even though he adamantly was opposed to accepting the ancient observations of Galen, he falls into the trap of mixing his observations with the bias of centuries of beliefs prior to his time.

Though he is aware that the venous supply to the left and right testes arise from different parts of the vena cava, he cannot help to note that the left side is "impure" because "… that vein which is offered to the left testis is believed to take its origin from the lower aspect of the vein which approaches the left kidney for reason that it may not carry the pure blood to the testis in the manner of the right vein but rather the serous blood, which by its salty and acrid quality may bring about an itching for the emission of the semen."

Vesalius' seminal errors are understandable and he was fully aware of the limitations of his knowledge and continuously advised his students to continue to observe and test his own findings.

Early life

Andreas Vesalius was born into a lineage of medical families in Brussels, Belgium, and has become known as the father of modern anatomy. He was the second son of Andries van Wessel and Isabel Crabbe, born at a quarter to six in the morning on 31 December 1514[1]. His youth appears to have been given in large part to his pursuit of the family tradition of medicine.

He was fortunate in that his family heritage was to serve the royalty of the Holy Roman Empire and they had managed to accumulate an impressive private library of medical classics. André, later Latinised to Andreas, learned Latin, Greek and Hebrew and followed the typical pathway to higher education. He matriculated to the school of his fathers, the University of Louvain at age 15, on 25 February 1530.

Developing his first medical mentor, Nicolaus Florenas encouraged his transfer to the University of Paris at the end of August 1533, at age 18[1]. Vesalius recounted that he had already managed to achieve some skill in anatomical dissection, obtaining numerous types of animals for this purpose (mice, doormice, cats and dogs)[2]. He had already read extensively the anatomical works of Galen and Avicenna.

From personal statements made by Andreas later in the "Letter on the China Root" we learn that his education there was something of a disappointment[3]. He continued to advance in dissection and became a prosector to one of his professors, Johann Guinter of Andernach.

In fact, Guinter acknowledged the talents of his young protégé in his first edition of his anatomical textbook in 1536. Guinter wrote of him "…a young man, by Hercules, of great promise, possessing an extraordinary knowledge

[1] O'Malley, C. D., *Andreas Vesalius of Brussels*. University of California Press: Berkeley, 1964.

[2] Tarshis, J. *Father of Modern Anatomy Andreas Vesalius*. The Dial Press: New York, 1969.

[3] Vesalius, A. *The Epitome of Andreas Vesalius*. Translated by L.R. Lind, Macmillan: New York, 1949.

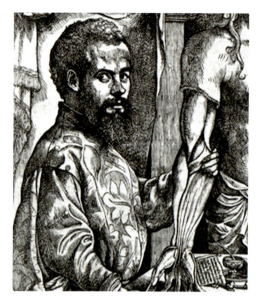

Figure 1: The original woodcut illustration of the only known image of Andreas Vesalius from the *Epitome*.

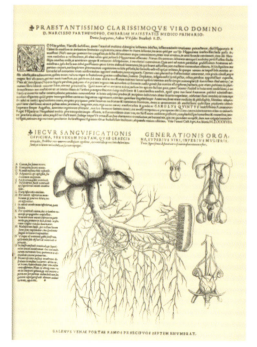

Figure 2: Genitourinary illustrations from *Tabulae sex*.

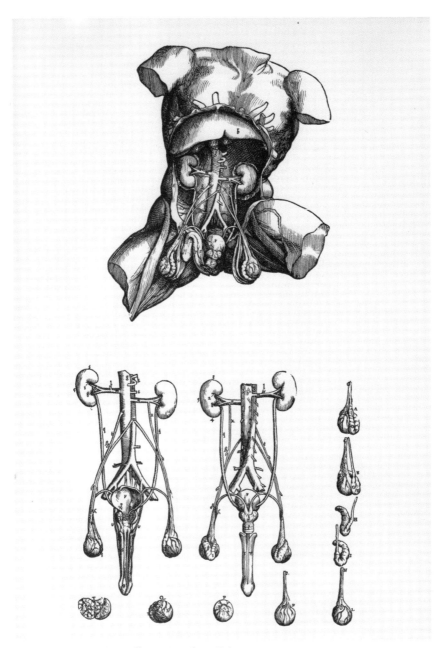

Figure 3: Genitourinary illustrations from *Epitome*.

of medicine, learned in both languages, and very skilled in dissection of bodies[2]."

A magnum opus

Vesalius' *magnum opus* was finally published in Basel, Switzerland by his friend Johannes Oporinus. Vesalius spared no expense in the creation of his work. He had worked assiduously for five years preparing for all aspects of this work. He had carefully worked with the artists and complained about the difficulties in working with some of them. This is one of the several lingering mysteries regarding this work, who were the artist(s)?[4]

The illustrations are performed by the studio of the master painter of Venice, Titian, but who deserves actual credit may never be entirely clear. The wood blocks were cut from pear wood, against the grain and treated with linseed oil.[5] These were then packed carefully for the trans-Alpine cross to Basel. The *De humani corporis fabrica libri septum* was dedicated to the emperor Charles V on 1 August 1542. The colophon displayed the date of June 1543.

The book was a magnificent testament to the vision of this young physician (Fig. 1). It was folio-sized with 636 pages and 73 plates. The portrait of Vesalius was present depicting him dissecting the arm of a woman. In addition, it had a magnificent title page that itself was a masterpiece laden with much symbolism.

He used ornate and illustrated capital letters that also bore anatomical themes. The *Fabrica* consists of seven books- skeleton (1), muscles (2), vascular system (3), nervous system (4), abdominal viscera and organs of reproduc-

[4] Saunders, J.B. DeC.M., O'Malley, C.D. *The Illustrations from the Works of Andreas Vesalius of Brussels.* World: New York, 1850.

[5] Cushing, H. *A Bio-Bibliography of Andreas Vesalius.* Henry Schuman: New York, 1943.

tion (5), thoracic viscera (6), and the brain (7).[4] The *Fabrica* was completed by Vesalius at the age of 28 and there is evidence that he worked upon this for five years.

Two months later, Vesalius published the smaller companion piece from the same publisher called simply the *Epitome*. This was released with both Latin and German translations and is dedicated to Prince Philip, son of Charles V and king of Spain. It consisted of 14 folio pages measuring 21 by 16 inches with 11 anatomical plates.

The unique thing about the *Epitome* was a human figure that measures 42.5 cm in height which was meant to be a cut-out figure for anatomical overlay. The Epitome is both a descriptive anatomy and an atlas. Vesalius himself, called this work an appendix, index, compendium and a pathway to the *Fabrica*.

A modern anatomist

The *Epitome* also differs from the *Fabrica* in terms of gross layout. There are only six books in the *Epitome* - bones and cartilages (1), muscles and ligaments (2), abdominal viscera (3), thoracic viscera and vascular system (4), the brain and nervous system (5), and organs of reproduction (6)[4]. Again, the *Epitome* was not repetitive and should be considered a book in its own right. His style was clear and brief. He assumed a more authoritative tone and was condensing his ideas. He obviously was trying to avoid any of the philosophical implications that his work was at odds with classic teachings.

Review of both published works is readily available to students of Vesaliana because of recent English translations both in print and on the internet[6,7]. In addition, numerous authors have begun to scrutinise his writings. The work of Andreas Vesalius constitutes one of the greatest treasures of Western civilisation and Sir William Osler noted that he was "the first modern anatomist to place his study on a firm foundation of observation[8]."

He states that his book was "not only the foundation of modern Medicine as a science, but the first positive achievement of science itself in modern times[8]." Most people are generally aware of Vesalius and his anatomical drawings, few can clearly express the true magnitude of his achievements.

This study was intended to review the genitourinary anatomy and place it into context of the overall work. This particular investigation is concerned with Vesalius' *Epitome* chapter VI "Concerning the Organs Which Minister To the Propagation of the Species" and the *Fabrica* Plates 58 & 59 regarding the urinary tract. This represents a review of his statements and anatomical descriptions of the genitourinary system.

Perpetuating misconceptions

Vesalius was aware that there were errors in his work, especially in books 3-5. He always intended to return to these areas after further research. Much has been written about the inaccuracies of the female genital anatomy, but little has been mentioned about his male genital errors[9-12].

Focusing upon the first illustrations of *Tabulae Sex*, the male genital anatomy shows

6
Vesalius, A. *De humani corporis fabrica libri septum*. Book V. Jeremy Norman, 2008.

7
http://vesalius.northwestern.edu/

8
Osler, W. *The Collected Essays of Sir William Osler*.Volume II. McGovern and Roland (Eds.). Gryphon Editions: New York, 1996, pp. 63-66.

9
Ball, J.M. *Andreas Vesalius, the Reformer of Anatomy*. Medical Science Press: St.Louis, 1910.

10
Singer, C. *A Short History of Anatomy from the Greeks to Harvey*. 2nd edition. Dover: New York, 1957.

11
Toedo-Perevra, L.H. "De Humani Corporis Fabrica surgical revolution". *J Invest Surg*. 2008. 21(5):232-6.

12
Vons, J. "Epitome, an ignored work of Andreas Vesalius". *Hist Sci Med*. 2006. 40(2):177-89.

anatomically correct vasculature, but the prostate was atypical, the seminal vesicles were absent, and the penis was sigmoid all typical of canine anatomy (Figs. 2-4). Vesalius did announce to the reader that animals were used in some instances.

In the *Epitome*, the anatomy was the same and he admitted to being the artist of these illustrations. Here, in the text he described the impurity of the L-sided male reproductive structures, because the venous blood supply descends from the renal vein. This makes the left side inferior to that of the right side.

In this he was simply perpetuating Galenic misconceptions:
> But that vein is offered to the left testis is believed to take its origin from the lower aspect of the vein which approaches the left kidney for reason that it may not carry the pure blood to the testis in the manner of the right vein but rather the serous blood, which by its salty and acrid quality may bring about an itching for emission of semen[4].

Though priding himself on his observational skills, he could not help falling into the Aristotelian dogmatism that also plagued Galen.

Vesalius had begun to doubt much of the anatomical and perhaps some of the functional observations that had held sway of the medical profession for a millennium and a half. He openly declared to those interested that there was much more work to do!

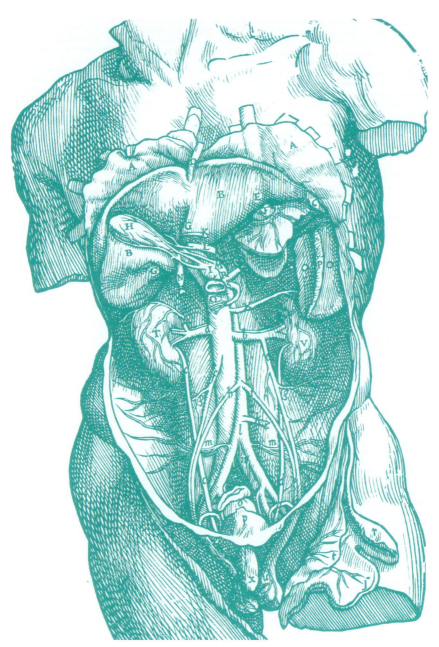

Figure 4: Genitourinary illustrations from *De fabrica*.

13
Androutsos, G. "The urology in the anatomical plates of Andreas Vesalius (1514-1564)". *Prog Urol*. 2005. 15(3):544-50.

14
DeBroe, M.E., Sacre, D., Snelders, E.D., De Weerdt, D.L. "The Flemish anatomist Andreas Vesalius (1514-1564) and the kidney". *Am J Nephrol*. 1997. 17:3-4:252-60.

After 12 years, he finally returned to Oporinus for a second, revised edition of *Fabrica*, in 1555[5]. He was more organised then, having more experience. The pages were thicker, the type was more legible, and some of the woodcuts were improved. Yet, male genitourinary anatomy remained uncorrected[13]. He had not found the seminal vesicles, and the fine vascular anatomy was lacking. He was on the cusp of discovering circulation, but could not make the leap!

Five generations of Vesalian anatomists would follow in his wake, making great strides in furthering his legacy of anatomical and physiological observation.[14] The fourth post- Vesalian chair of anatomy, Fabricius, would have a pupil that would finally make the next truly great observation, the circulation of blood by William Harvey[10].

A monumental achievement

Andreas Vesalius (1514-1565) produced a monumental achievement by placing anatomy and surgery back within the realm of science. He taught his pupils to question authority, to observe independently, and to perform "hands on" research for themselves. That was the main legacy of this remarkable individual and he never claimed to have finished his work in human anatomy.

His message had its outspoken critics, however, anyone with integrity and desire now had an open door to further advance mankind's knowledge of development, disease, and therapeutics. That Vesalius understood this is quite evident from his other surviving writings, the "Letter on the China Root": "Then, and not until then, could they accurately consider the points in question, and could impartially weigh the issues that were set forth with utmost candor and with the primary purpose of furthering investigation[4]."

His final published work, in 1561, *An Examination of Gabriele Fallopio's Anatomic Observations* he praised his heirs effort and extended his beliefs in scientific medicine even further.[5]

So much Vesaliana discussed the anatomy illustrations only, comparing the manuscript that rivals daVinci's *Mona Lisa* as a masterpiece of the Renaissance[15]. Within the cradle of early modern science, 1543 was the *annus mirabilis* which was made singular by the publication of two sentinel works, *De revolutionibus orbium coelestium libri sex* by the physician Nicolaus Copernicus and the *De humani corporis fabrica libri septum* by fellow Paduan physician, Andreas Vesalius.

[15] Moran, M.E. "The da Vinci robot". *J Endourol*. 2006. 20(12):986-990.

The former lifted the hooded veil of subservience to the great classical thinkers and began to question and evaluate nature using observation by his own senses. With new observations revealing unexpected findings, these nascent philosophers of new sciences began to boldly extrapolate their own implications. They opened the doors to their students and their student's students to ultimately improve mankind's understanding.

Anatomy from 1543 onwards would now be a vital part of medical education and set the stage for the realignment of surgery and surgeons with the ancient profession. Vesalius' spark kindled a flame poised to explode from the curiosity of men and women. In France, Amboise Paré became an ardent early proponent as did students in Padua, Pisa, Bologna and Rome!

By the time of the second edition of the *Fabrica*, in 1555, there were very few nay-sayers left, and at the home of enlightened academic freedom, Padua, the first two disciples were already advancing the frontiers of knowledge; Realdus Columbus and Gabriel Fallopius followed and disseminated the master's message. Some were even questioning the Aristotelian/Galenic humoural theories of disease. The floodgates had been breached and medicine never again would be arrested by the empiric dogma that stymied progress for 15 centuries.

After five generations of anatomists, the male genital anatomy would finally become whole, and even the names and detailed vasculature of the pelvis would fall to the Vesalian heir, Fabricius. His rival at Bologna, Malpighi would complete renal anatomy until circulation was given to physicians by the Fabrician pupil, William Harvey.

The cascade to modern urological anatomy and physiology can be seen by the Dutch physician, Jan van Beverwyck who almost immediately wrote a book on stone disease incorporating the most up-to-date physiology into a new theory of stone formation, inserting the importance of circulation to the kidneys[16]. Vesalius concluded his magnum opus by humbly stating "Farewell, and use these, my efforts, as frankly as they are offered," and use them they did. *Ocyus, iucunde et tuto*.

16
Van Beverwyck, J. *De calculo renum et vesicae liber singularis. Cum epistolis et consultationibus magnorum virorum*. Leiden, 1638.

Correspondence to:
Michael E. Moran
Southwest Urology
1100 N. Eldorado Pl. Tucson, AZ 34990
E-mail: memoran2@juno.com

THE LEGEND OF SUN SHIMIAO: THE MAN WHO INVENTED URETHRAL CATHETERISATION

Wei Wang and Peter M. Thompson

Department of Urology, Beijing Tongren Hospital, Capital Medical University, Beijing, China, and Department of Urology, King's Collge Hospital, King's College, London, UK.

Department of Urology, King's Collge Hospital, King's College, London, UK.

1
Zheng, B.C. "The King of Medicine: Sun Simiao". *Journal of Traditional Chinese Medicine*. 1986. 6:210-211.

2
Hsu, H.Y., Peacher, W.G. *Chen's History of Chinese Medical Science*. Modern Drug Publishers Co.: Taipei, Taiwan, 1977.

3
Unschuld, P.U. *Medical Ethics in Imperial China. A Study in Historical Anthropology*. University of California Press: Berkeley, CA, 1979.

4
Chen, P. *History and Development of Traditional Chinese Medicine*. Science Press: Beijing, 1999.

Sun Shimiao was a famous physician and taoist of the Sui and Tang dynasty (Fig. 1). He was titled as King of Medicine for his significant valued and varied contributions to the speciality of Chinese Traditional Medicine. The work he was most noted for was his two 30-volume works *A Thousand Gold for Emergencies* and his invention of urethral catherisation.[1,2] He is also known for the text *On the Absolute Sincerity of Great Physicians*, often called "the Chinese Hippocratic Oath", which is still required reading for Chinese physicians.[3]

Born in 581 A.D. at Huayuan (central area of ancient China), Sun was a sickly child, and the cost of medical treatments that reduced his family to poverty, motivated him to enter into the study of medicine. He rapidly learned the wisdom of Taoism, Confucianism and Buddhism, mastered the Chinese classics by age of 20, and quickly rose to fame for his apothecary skills. Although Sun Shimiao travelled distances as far as Sichuan province in search of medical knowledge and herbal prescriptions, he lived most of his life secluded in the caves of Wubai Mountain (Fig.2). Preferring the simplicity of a hermit's life, this great and humble physician spent his professional life treating all who was unfortunate enough to be stricken with disease (Fig. 3), and turned down official court positions that were offered to him by three successive Chinese emperors[4].

Sun wrote prodigiously, producing his famous 30-volume book *A Thousand Gold for Emergencies* that would establish his place as a central figure in the field of herbal medicine and acupuncture (Fig.4). This book, a classic text of prescriptions, significantly updated China's original medical treatise, the Neiching, which was put together around 100 B.C. The book presented life-saving remedies, hence the title reflecting their great value - a life is worth more than a thousand gold coins.[5] A mystical origin was attributed to some of the formulas, as with this story from the Song Dynasty (660-1279 A.D.): Sun Shimiao once saved the dragon of the Kunming Lake (in Yunnan Province) and, as a reward, got 30 magical recipes from the Dragon Palace (Fig.5).

A Thousand Gold for Emergencies was not merely a collection of formulas (of which there were an astonishing 4,500), but a treatise on medical practice that reviewed the work since the Han Dynasty (ca. 100 B.C.). Sun included treatises on acupuncture, herbal medicine, massage, diet, and exercises. So comprehensive in scope was this treatise that later authorities declared it the first encyclopaedia of clinical practice. So impressive were Sun's teachings that in the 10th century, they were incorporated into the famous Japanese medical text, the *Ishimpo*. A fundamental underpinning of Chinese medicine revolves around the twin forces of nature, yin and yang, whose balance is believed to be integral to a person's health. The legend of Sun Shimiao is a legend of commanding control of these forces. In paintings and other works of art, he is regularly featured showing a tiger (yin) below at his feet, and a dragon (yang) above in his outstretched hand (Fig. 6).

[5] State Administration of Traditional Chinese Medicine. *Advanced Textbook on Traditional Chinese Medicine and Pharmacology.* Vol. 1. New World Press: Beijing, 1995.

For the urologists, Sun should be best remembered for being the first to describe successful urethral catheterisation. Before Sun's time, patients with acute urinary retention were treated by acupuncture and herbal medicine. Unfortunately many of the patients still could not urinate. One afternoon, Sun saw a patient with acute urinary retention after failure of acupuncture. A child playing with spring onion caught his attention. He used the hollow leaves of spring onion as a catheter and passed it down the urethra of the patient. He was successful and the patient was able to pass urine through the hollow leaf and the retention was relieved (Fig. 7).[6] The mechanisms to explain this technique might be: use of air to dilate the urethra; relaxation of smooth muscle within the prostate and bladder neck; increased pressure within the bladder. After that, Chinese physicians began to use differed kinds of reeds and straws to perform urethral catheterisation. In 1036 CE, Avicenna described the first flexible catheter made from stiffened animal skins.[6]

The following are some of the many contributions by this great physician: that goitre in mountainous regions could be cured with seaweeds (which contain iodine) or with thyroid gland extracts from sheep and deer; that night blindness could be successfully treated with livers from oxen and sheep (vitamin A); and that beriberi is curable with unpolished rice which contains vitamin B. Sun also made significant contributions in ophthalmology and in women's health. In the beginning chapters of his book, he reasoned that special prescriptions were necessary for women because "they get pregnant, give birth and suffer from uterine damage," and estimated that women's disorders were "ten

6
Wang, W., Thompson, P. M. "Sun Shimiao: the man who invented urethral catheterization". *European Urology Supplements*. 2009. 8:162.

7
Du, Y. "A brief history of the application of urethral catheterization in ancient China". *Zhonghua Yi Shi Za Zhi*. 1995. 25:35-37.

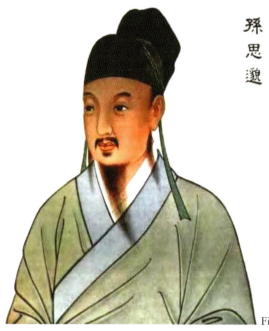

Figure 1: Sun Shimiao (581-682AD).

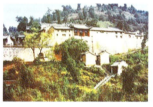

Figure 2: The former residence of Sun Shimiao, located in Yaoxian County of Shaanxi Province.

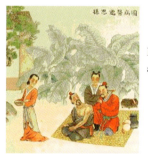

Figure 3: Sun Shimiao attending to a patient.

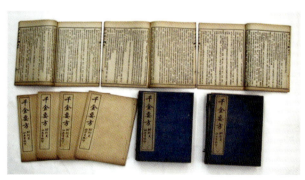

Figure 4: *A Thousand Gold for Emergencies*, Physician's reference book for emergency treatment.

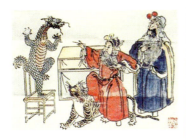

Figure 5: Curing dragon king with acupuncture.

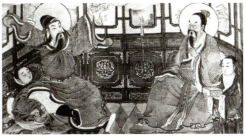

Figure 6: Sun had the power to keep the balance of Yin (the tiger) and Yang (the dragon).

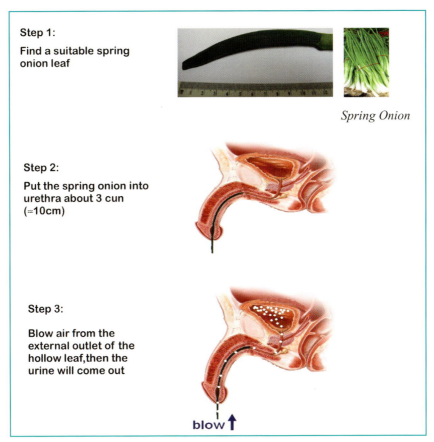

Step 1:

Find a suitable spring onion leaf

Spring Onion

Step 2:

Put the spring onion into urethra about 3 cun (≈10cm)

Step 3:

Blow air from the external outlet of the hollow leaf, then the urine will come out

blow ↑

Figure 7: Sun's spring onion catheterisation technique. All illustrations are based on Sun's book *A Thousand Gold for Emergencies*.

121

times more difficult to treat than those of males, perhaps because of yin influences (swelling and dampness)."[8]

If Hippocrates is ancient Greece's enduring legacy to Western medicine, then Sun Shimiao is ancient China's gift to the world of Eastern medicine. Despite being vastly separated by time (a thousand years), distance (the opposite end of the globe), and culture (Western vs. Eastern), these two giants bequeathed to the medical profession a common language of science and ethics.

Like Hippocrates, Sun believed that diseases resulted from the imbalances of natural forces, championed the use of dietary and herbal treatments, and wrote prodigiously. Most remarkably, he promulgated a code of conduct for the virtuous physician that captured many of the exhortations of the Hippocratic Oath, although it is virtually certain he had never heard of Hippocrates, much less been exposed to his teachings. Sun stated simply his belief of what the virtuous physician ought to do, and what he ought to refrain from doing. It is less of a formal code, and more of a reminder. Patient autonomy and physician truth-telling were not part of Sun's code - nor of the Hippocratic Oath. Instead, the main ethical principles focused on compassion, justice, beneficence, and humility. These values remain valid today, and define the ethical doctor. They are presented below in condensed[3,9]:

1. Look upon those who have come to grief as if he himself had been struck, and he should sympathise with them deep in his heart.
2. Do not give way to wishes and desires,

[8] Needham, J. *Science and Civilization in China*. Vol. 5, No. 2. Cambridge University Press: London, 1974.

[9] Tan, S.Y. "Medicine in Stamps Sun Si Miao (581-682 A.D.): China's pre-eminent physician". *Singapore Med J*. 2002. 43:224-225.

but develop first a marked attitude of compassion.
3. Do not ponder over his own fortune or misfortune and thus preserve life and have compassion for it.
4. Whoever suffers from abominable things, such as ulcers or diarrhoea, will be looked upon with contempt by people. Yet even in such cases, an attitude of compassion, of sympathy, and of care should develop; by no means should there arise an attitude of rejection.
5. Treat all patients alike, whether powerful or humble, rich or poor, old or young, beautiful or ugly, resentful relatives or kind friends, Chinese nationals or foreigners, fools or wise men.
6. Neither dangerous mountain passes nor the time of day, neither weather conditions nor hunger, neither thirst nor fatigue, should keep him from helping whole-heartedly.
7. Make a dignified appearance, neither luminous nor sombre.
8. It is not permissible to be talkative and make provocative speeches, to make fun of others and raise one's voice, to decide right from wrong, and to discuss other people and their business.
9. The wealth of others should not be the reason to prescribe precious and expensive drugs, and thus make access to help more difficult and underscore one's own merits and abilities. Such conduct has to be regarded as contrary to the teaching of magnanimity. The object is to help.

10. It is inappropriate to emphasise one's reputation, to belittle the rest of physicians, and to praise one's own virtue. Indeed, in actual life someone who has accidentally healed a disease then strides around with his head raised, shows conceit, and announces that no one in the entire world could measure up to him. In this respect, all physicians are evidently incurable!

Sun Shimiao is of course one of the most interesting figures in the history of Chinese traditional medicine. It is not too difficult to support this judgment, even though biographical details of this Tang physician are only fragmentary. In his lifetime, Sun Shimiao was a famous clinician; to posterity, he left voluminous formularies that have been influential until the present.[10]

10 Unschuld, P.U. *Medicine in China: Historical Artifacts and Images*. Prestel Verlag: Munich, 2000.

Correspondence to:
Wei Wang
Urology Department
Beijing Tongren Hospital
Capital Medical University
1 Dongjiaominxiang Street
Dongcheng District
Beijing 100730, China
E-mail: medtrip@gmail.com

THE "ORIENTAL TESTIS": A SHORT HISTORY

S.N. Cenk Buyukunal, Ayten Altıntaş

Department of Pediatric Surgery Urology, Cerrahpaşa Medical Faculty, University of Istanbul, Turkey.

Department of History of Medicine and Medical Ethics, Cerrahpaşa Medical Faculty, University of Istanbul, Turkey.

The testis, as an organ of power, fertility and masculinity, has been mentioned in many communities, civilisations and legends throughout the history of mankind. In the ancient tribes of the Turks, Mesopotamia, Ottoman Empire and Islamic civilisation, the testis has always been regarded as the "symbol organ" of power and fertility. In this study the aim is to present small passages from various medical historical documents and provide a brief history of how the testis is regarded in the world's Oriental regions.

Castration in antiquity

Castration practised on animals and humans has a long history and dates back to prehistoric times. In antiquity the male animals domesticated and used in tillage had to be castrated as they were often unruly and wild. In the course of time, castration methods for animals have undergone changes. In the caves of Mesopotamia, where there is evidence of human presence from the prehistoric age, it is possible to find castrated bull figures which proves the existance of castration procedures.

In what used to be old Babylon, archeaologists found texts related to the castration of bulls mentioned in the Laws of Hammurabi (2200 B.C.). In ancient Egyptian civilisation castrated bulls were used in farming and agriculture. On the other hand, castration was strictly forbidden in the Old Testament. In P3, Chapter 22 it was mentioned that "you should never sacrifice castrated animals in the name of God and never let other people do that!"

However, even in the early days of Judaism, the Israelis practised different castration techniques in various animals such as squeezing the testicle by hand or by using a special hammer, tortion and pulling.

In the 4th century A.D. of the Byzantine Empire, official veterinerians practised the castration of horses. The famous collection called *Hippiatrika* includes various written documents of cavaliers and official veterinerians of Byzantine army and contains texts of castration.[1,2]

The ancient Turkish tribes Hien-un and Hun-ok also practised castration in horses in the belief that these horses will be quicker and faster (2200 B.C.). These animals were called *equus hunnicus* by the Romans.

According to the first Turkish Dictionary written in the 11th century by Mahmut of Kasgar (original name: Divan-ı Lugat-it-Turk), castration is mentioned as *argılamak, enemek.* And a method said to be one of the oldest known to the Turkish tribes was "castration by teeth." The procedure was very simple and effective. The male animal was pinned to the ground down by the castrator and the testicular vessels were squeezed between his clenched teeth[1,3].

Castration in Islam

In Islamic religion the act of castration was strictly forbidden both in humans and animals. However "castration procedure " has been mentioned in all Arabic veterinarian textbooks published since the 9th century[1,2]. In the book

[1] Altintas, A. "Testicular hormons and anabolizing hormones in history of medicine." *Thesis for Medical History and Ethics*, Cerrahpasa Medical Faculty: Istanbul, 1982.

[2] Göyünç, N. "Castration". In: *Encyclopedia of Islam*, Vol. 12/1. Istanbul, 1977, p. 66.

[3] Altıntaş, A. "Castration by teeth among the Turks". *Folklore and Etnography Studies*. Istanbul, 1984, pp. 13-15.

Management of Horses written by Ibn Ahi Hizam (9th century), in Chapter 13 there is a passage that says: "...the castration of horses is religiously forbidden, but it is necessary..."

One of the most important writers of late 12th century was Ibn-ul Avvam from Andalucia, Spain. In the last part of his book *Kitab-al Falaha* (Chapter 34) he mentioned the castration of pigeons, ducks and roosters. He advised the castration of rooster which he said will result to "a better meat."

Abd Al Mumin Al-Dimyati (1217-1306) was born in south-east Anatolia and later lived in Egypt. In his famous book *Kitab Fadl al-Hayl* "Grace of Horses" he described the castration procedure for horses (Chapter 2).

Castration techniques

Ebu Bekr was one of the most famous veterinerians of the Islamic world during the 15th to the 16th centuries. In his veterinary textbook he mentioned castration as a "religiously forbidden technique." But he also declared the benefits of castration in some animals.

The four major castration techniques that he advised were as follows: cutting by thermal coagulation; cutting by using a scalpel; squeezing and the kaso technique. The kaso was a popular technique and in this procedure, the *funniculus spermaticus* was clipped by using two wooden clips, after which a hemostasis orchiectomy procedure was performed. Clips were left in situ for a couple of days and the scrotal wound was protected against infection with a local application of sulfur compounds[1].

Castration in humans

In prehistoric ages it was customary to take out the testicles of defeated enemies. When two tribes clashed, the victors cut off the testicles of young boys from the defeated tribe, destroying their reproductive capacity. Thus, those who survived the bloody battles could only live as eunuchs.

In Babylon, 2000 B.C., castration was a kind of routine surgical procedure for ill-looking and weak male children. According to the historical texts of the Mesopotamian region, during the time of King Hammurabi castration was performed by barbers as well as other minor surgical procedures [1,2,4].

Queen Semiramis, the famous Asurian queen and wife of king Ninus, was recorded to be the first who used castrated slaves in the harem. The aim was to protect the queen and other women of the palace from the complications of illetigimate sexual relations.

During the reign of the Pharoahs in Egyptian civilisation, castration was a type of religious and legal punishment for Egyptian citizens who were accused of sexual assaults. This procedure was also used in punishing the enemies of Egypt. During the reign of the Hittite Emperor Hattushilish-I (1650-1600 B.C.), slaves were castrated according to the orders of the emperor, implying that the Hittites already knew that the testicles are organs for fertilisation.

In the Saga of Gilgamis, there was an account of the violent struggle between Kumarbi and Anu, which ended with Kumarbi tearing up and eating Anu's testicles[1,2,3,4] (Fig. 1). And in

4
Buyukunal, S.N.C., Altintas, A. "History of oriental testis". *EAU History of Urology Meeting*, Medical Museum, Vienna, 2005.

Instanbul during the Byzantine period, castrated robust slaves were very popular among aristocrat ladies and were used to satisfy the sexual desires of their masters. Obviously having sexual relations with the eunuch slaves carry no risks of pregnancy.

Eunuchs also occupied or played key roles in the military. One of the most famous generals of Emperor Justinien, commandor Narses (644 A.D.), was a eunuch. And during Emperor Kislave's reign there were a number of famous generals and high-rankling officials who were in charge of the Byzantine palace.

Castratis in the arts

Castratis as church choir members was known in Istanbul during the Byzantine Empire, and the most difficult solo parts were often performed by castratis. This tradition also became popular in the Roman Catholic Church during the 17th century. The Byzantine Emperor Constantin the Great (274-337 A.D.), however, was strongly against castration and was the founder of the "Penalties Against Castration." Despite the edict eunuch slaves as 'gifts' were highly appreciated by some Byzantine Emperors such as Leo III Isauricus (717-744 A.D.)

According to the Greek Historian Heredotes, some of the high rankling officials of the Iranian palace were selected from the ranks of eunuchs (1). In the textbook of Paulus Aegina (625-690 A.D.), the technical details of castration as a surgical procedure have been mentioned in details. Haly Abbas (930-994 A.D.) translated this book into Arabic.

During the medieval period some regions in North Africa and France widely practised cas-

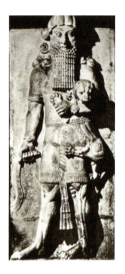

Figure 1: The violent struggle between Kumarbi and Anu ended with Kumarbi tearing up and eating Anu's testicles.

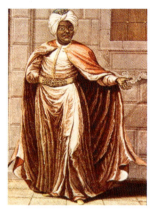

Figure 2: *Harem agasi* means "chief of the Harem" and he was one of the high rankling officials in Ottoman Palace.

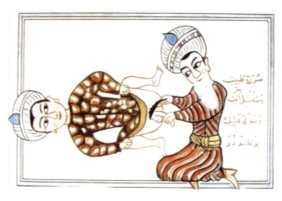

Figure 3: A castration procedure. Sabuncuoglu, 15th century.

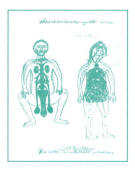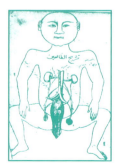

Figures 4 a,b: *Pictured Anatomy Book* describes the anatomical details of the testis, ductus, epididimis and vasculature-like attachments of the testis.

tration. Nearly 35,000 children per year from North Africa, Ethiophia and Sudan were bought as slaves. Only a very small amount of money was paid for each child (nearly two US dollars). These children were later castrated in Arne region, city of Verdun in France and Ghebel-Eter and Abou-Gerhe in Egypt. Around 33% to 75% of these children died during or just after the procedure mainly due to bleeding and complications. For that reason, the final price paid for each eunuch child after the completion of all procedures was much higher than the initial payment (nearly two thousand US dollars)[4].

Castration in the Ottoman Period

Castration is prohibited in the Islamic civilisation and the shariah. The employment of eunuchs in the service of the palace started under Muaviye (660-680 A.D.). Thereafter they were employed by the Abbasis, the Samanids, the Gazneans, Selcuks, Ilhanids, Fatimis and the Islamised Mongol states [1,2].

The famous Arabic physician Albucasis (Zahrawi) from Cordoba in Andalucia, described castration techniques in his textbook *Kitab al Tasrif*, written in the 10th century. These techniques included squeezing (risk of surviving testicular tissue!), open surgical technique, the incision of scrotum, clamping the testicular vessels and excision of the gonad[6,7].

In the famous textbook *El-Kanun Fi't Tıb, "Law of Medicine"*, written by Avicenna (Ibn-i Sina, 11th century), the anatomical description of the organ was given in detail. To quote: ".... there are four types of muscles and they all surround and cover the testicle. Cremaster and dartos muscles protect each testicle and enhances the mobility of the organ"[8].

6
Buyukunal, S.N.C., Sari, N. "Serafeddin Sabuncuoğlu, the author of the earliest pediatric surgical atlas: Cerrahiye-i Ilhaniye". *J Pediatr Surg*. 1991. 26:1148-1151.

7
Zahravi, Kitab Al Taşrif. Chap. 30, f:39. From the *Collection of Haci Beşir* Aga. Suleymaniye Library, Istanbul.

8
İbn-i Sina. *El-Kanun Fi't-Tıbb*. Book 1. Translated by Kahya, E. Vol.103 (5). Atatürk Cultural Center: Ankara, 1995, p. 67.

Castration was strictly forbidden by the Ottoman empire. However, eunuchs who were brought from Africa (mainly Egypt) were highly appreciated by the palace, especially by the members of the harem. The employment of eunuchs in the Ottoman palace begun during Sultan Murat-II's reign (1421-1444). The black eunuchs were in charge of the maintenance and protection of the harem[5,9]. These eunuchs, bought from slave traders coming from Northern Africa, Sudan and Egypt (Fig. 2), were presented as the gifts by the Ottoman officials of Egypt.

Damat Ali Pasha, the first Ottoman prime minister (1703-1730) tried to prevent castration by imposing legal and monetary penalties. However, after his assassination the practice continued albeit in a limited scale and until the abolition of the sultanate[5].

In the Ottoman Empire castration was a banned operation. But the details of the operation have been given in detail in major textbooks. Serafeddin Sabuncuoglu was one of the most important physicians of the 15th century, and in his well known textbook Cerrahiye-i Ilhaniye, (part 2, chapter 69, pp:109 a-b) he described an orchiectomy operation in detail. He mentioned: "As a student of medicine, you should know that castration is prohibited by religion. However in order not to miss any surgical procedure, we wanted to give some details of the procedure..."[6,10]

The author described two techniques:

1. Squeezing the testis in warm water until it becomes loose and almost impalpable.
2. Ligation of the pedicle and incising the

9
Dizdaroğlu, N. "Chief Black Eunuchs in the Ottoman History," Thesis from Literature Faculty, Istanbul University, Istanbul, 1948.

5
Altintaş, A. "Castration in medical practice during the Ottoman Empire". In: Kelami, A., Sari, N., Zülfikar, B., Altintas, A., Barlas, U., Özcan, A. (contrb.). *Art and Andrology*. Istanbul, 1992, pp. 121-125.

10
Verit, A., Aksoy, S. ,Kafalı, H., Verit, F.F. "Urologic techniques of Serafeddin Sabuncuoğlu in the 15th century Ottoman period". *Urology*. 2003. 62:776-778.

dartos layer and taking the testis out of scrotum. This was the procedure of choice since there will be no testicular remnants in both scrotal pouches. Bilateral orchiectomy has been performed as a two-stage operation. Sometimes penectomy is added as a third stage procedure(!) (Fig. 3)

In the anatomy textbook of Semseddin-i Itaki (17th century) the anatomical specialities of testis has been described in detail[1,11]:
a) The testis has four different muscle layers;
b) Sperm is manifactured in the testis and the ejaculate is the ultimate distillation of blood;
c) The whitish color of testis resembles the color of the ejaculate; and
d) The anatomical details of ductus and epididimis were stated and the importance of the ductus in sperm transportation of sperm was also described (Fig.4 a,b).

Other interesting remarks from the same chapter were:
- The male ejaculate determines the spirit of the fetus. The liquids coming from the female genital organ form the somatic part of the fetus.
- The testis collects the blood coming from the kidneys. This blood is processed in the testis and gains its white color, and this liquid may create a new organism. Details of the new organism is "...decided by the God."

Organotherapy/orotherapy

This is a different type of treatment modality for impotency. The testis tissue itself or testicular tissue suspensions were used for this purpose. According to a translation of the Eber papyrus from Egypt (1550 B.C.) impotence

11
Şemseddin-i Itaki. *Pictured Anatomy Book*,1630. Translated by Kahya. E. Atatürk Cultural Center Publications, Ankara, 1996, pp. 221-223.

was treated by using "...a mixture of testicular extracts..." from bear, horse, fox, donkey, goat, pig, wild rabbit and deer.

In ancient China similar problems were treated by using powder from goat testis. In India, the compound powder of crocodile, rat, frog and bird testes was used for the treatment of erectile disorders. In Islamic time and the Ottoman Empire some other organotherapy modalities were recommended by authorities such as the following:
- Yuhanna Ibn Musavach (777-857) used a mixture of blended camel and horse testes in donkey's milk;
- In the book (Firdausu'l Hikmet) of Rabban-Al Tabari (850) the use of deer testes was mentioned;
- Ibn Baytar in the 13th century advised men to eat a young bull's testes to cure erection problems; and
- Mustafa Fevzi Efendi in the 17th century advised taking the powder of dried deer testis to achieve proper erection.[1,4,12]

12
Altintas, A. "Aphrodisiac prescriptions mentioned in the Ottoman manuscripts on medicine dating from 17th and 18th centuries." In: Kelami, A. Sari, N., Zülfikar, B., Altintas, A., Barlas, U., Özcan, A. (contrb.). *Art and Andrology*. Istanbul,1992, pp. 85-91.

A deadly practice

Castration was the first-known surgical procedure on human testis. In ancient times at the end of bloody battles, it is customary to cut off the testicles of the members of defeated tribes and enemies. In the Orient the purpose of "castration" was somewhat different from the Western world and castration was apparently practiced in order to present eunuchs to the palaces of rulers and emperors.

Orchiectomy was strictly forbidden in Islamic religion and in the Eastern world. However, all major surgical textbooks contained details of this operation. Old veterinarian and medical textbooks mentioned the anatomy and physiology of the organ and provided technical details of various castration procedures.

Castration in childhood was a dangerous operation and mortality rates were high. This procedure was one of the black and shameful memories of mankind and should be seen or considered as a form of physical child abuse in the annals of ancient medicine.

Correspondence to:
S.N. Cenk Buyukunal
Park Maya sitesi A2 Blok No16, 34335
Akatlar-Istanbul Turkey
E-mail: cbuyukunal@tnn.net

THE RELATIONSHIP BETWEEN THE PHYSICIAN AND THE INSTRUMENT MAKER

As seen from the conflict between Jean Leroy d'Etiolles and Joseph-Frédéric Benoît Charrière

Michaela Zykan

International Nitze-Leiter Research Society of Endoscopy, Vienna, Austria.

Hic manus et oculus - "here hand and eye" - is an old saying of Swiss surgeons which could be interpreted in different ways: practice has to go hand in hand with science or skill has to be combined with theory. This motto can equally also be applied when looking at the history of medicine. In investigating various theories in the development of medical science, one should not neglect the practical medicine with all its auxiliary resources, which have all contributed to the best possible treatment of the patient[1]. This article therefore attempts to look closer into the relationship of those two poles - on the one hand the physician as the representative of the discipline who is aware of the medical issues and who may even have some idea how to tackle the difficulty; and on the other hand - the instrument maker who is able to bring the idea into reality.

With Philipp Bozzini's publication of the "Light conductor" in 1805, the era of endoscopy had begun - from that time onwards physicians in cooperation with their instrument makers constantly worked on technical improvements of endoscopic instruments in order to solve the inevitable problems of light, optics and handling.

[1] Boschung, U. "Chirurgiemechanik im 18. Jahrhundert". In: *Geschichte der Medizin und der medizinischen Technik*. Folge 8, 1980.

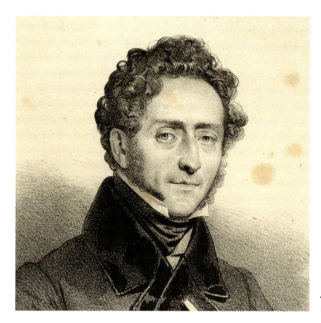

Figure 1:
Jacques Joseph Leroy
d'Etiolles (1798-1860).

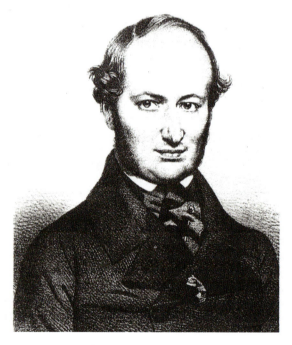

Figure 2:
Joseph-Frédéric Benoît
Charrière (1803-1876).

In view of its excellent surgeons and skilful instrument makers, Paris had become a centre for endoscopic development as of the first half of the 19th century.

In the history of the development of lithotripsy, the names of two French surgeons stand out. Jean Civiale (1796-1867) and Jean Jacques Joseph Leroy d'Etiolles (1798-1860) (Fig. 1) both worked on methods of removing stones from the bladder without submitting the patient to lithotomy. A bitter argument erupted between Leroy and Civiale as to who first conceived the idea of a lithotrite. Both spent a great deal of time claiming priority of invention and in defaming each other. It reached such proportions that the French Academy of Sciences appointed a commission to investigate. In 1831 it decided against Civiale, but two years later reversed that decision[2].

Frédéric Benoît Charrière (Fig. 2) was one of the best known instrument makers in Paris at the time.

Charrière was also actively involved in the development of lithotrity. The trilabe which was presented by Jean Civiale in 1824 was produced in his workshop. Among his other clients were surgeons like Pierre Solomon Ségalas (1792-1875), Jean Zulemie Amussat (1796-1856), le Baron Charles Louis Stanislas Heurteloupe (1791-1861), and Jean August Mercier (1811-1882). All those surgeons seemed to work in constant competition against each other in order to develop modifications to improve the handling and effectiveness of the instrumentation used in the urogenital tract.

2

Boschung, U. "Joseph-Frédéric-Benoit Charrière (1803-1876): Paris Surgical Instrument Maker from Switzerland". *Schweizerische Rundschau für Medizin*. 1985.74, 8:181-184.

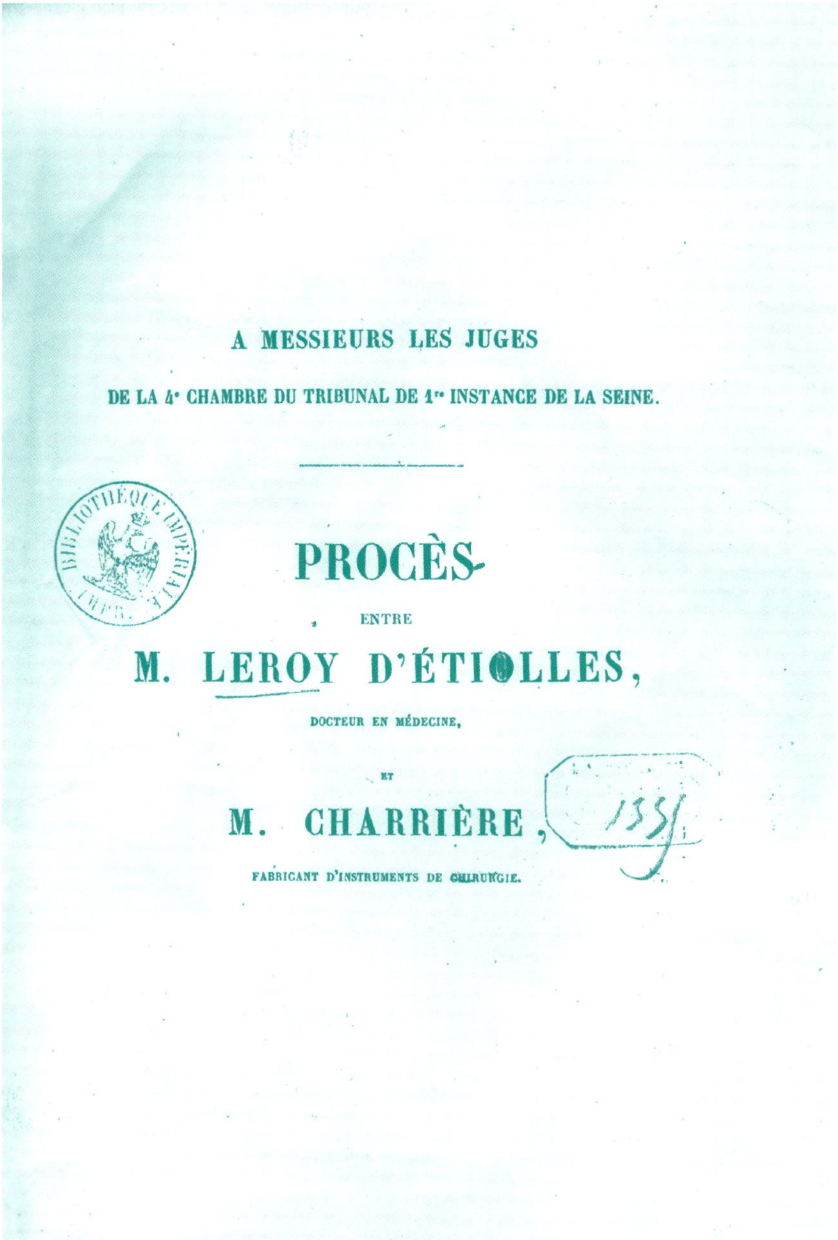

A MESSIEURS LES JUGES

DE LA 4ᵉ CHAMBRE DU TRIBUNAL DE 1ʳᵉ INSTANCE DE LA SEINE.

PROCÈS

ENTRE

M. LEROY D'ÉTIOLLES,

DOCTEUR EN MÉDECINE,

ET

M. CHARRIÈRE,

FABRICANT D'INSTRUMENTS DE CHIRURGIE.

Figure 4: Front page of the lawsuit of Leroy'Etiolles against B. Charrière.

Born in 1803 in Switzerland, Joseph-Frédéric Benoît Charrière moved to Paris at the age of 13 to work as an apprentice cutler. In 1820 he took over his master's workshop. The crucial stage of his career dates from his introduction to Guillaume Dupuytren, chief surgeon at the Hôtel Dieu hospital in Paris. Under Dupuytren's patronage, Charrière's business prospered and around 1825, 19 out of 20 surgeons consigned to him the fabrication of their working instruments, as well as their experimental ones (Fig. 3).

At the 1834 exposition of national industry, Charrière received his first medal to be followed by innumerable other distinctions. Although Charrière had become head of the largest and most important surgical instrument making company he got involved in disputes which led him to a number of court cases[3].

The following illustration from a plaint documents the turbulent relationship between Jean Leroy d'Etiolles and his instrument maker Joseph-Frédéric B. Charrière (Fig. 4).

What had happened between the instrument maker Charrière and the surgeon Leroy d'Etiolles who worked in a fruitful cooperation for over 20 years? After several years of disputes with his instrument maker, Leroy d'Etiolles finally decided to break up his cooperation with Charrière. Financial differences were among of the main reasons why the surgeon launched this complaint: Charrière's financial claims were not acceptable to him even though Charrière at the time still owed him several instruments which were supposed to serve as models for Charrière's work. Furthermore, d'Etiolles accused Charrière of not having kept accurate financial records:

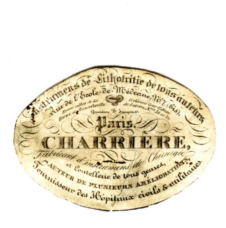

Figure 3:
Charrière's company label.

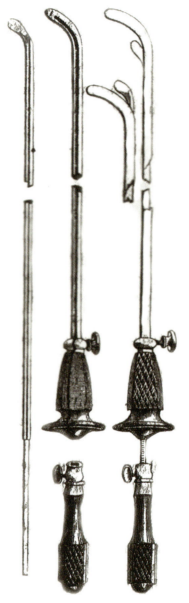

Figure 5:
The incisor by
Leroy d'Etiolles.

"les erreurs ne proviennent que d'un desordre dans ses ecritures".

Apart from the financial aspect the surgeon raised a second reason for his plaint: this concerned Charrière's disloyal behaviour towards him. Leroy d'Etiolles had invented a number of lithotrity instruments as well as other urological and surgical instruments which were subsequently made by Charrière according to the surgeon's precise instructions: "These instruments were my own creation but were also sold in the name of Frédéric Benoît Charrière to his other clients." Heated discussions with other surgeons were the consequence of this behaviour: The case of an improvement on a lithotriptor to facilitate the stone destruction made by d'Etiolle had initiated a first conflict with Jean Civiale. After careful examination of both instruments in 1836, the Academy of Sciences in Paris came to the conclusion that "it is possible that both lithotritists had the same idea but there is no doubt that Mr. Leroy d'Etiolles was the first one who added this improvement."

Moreover Charrière was accused of having exhibited and demonstrated this particular improvement as his own at the universal exposition in London, in 1851. As we know, the universal exposition in London had contributed significantly to Charrière's success. The *Gazette des hopitaux* reported on the improvement of the mechanism of the lithotriptor introduced by Mr. Charrière and praised him for it. The big success at the London universal exhibition undoubtedly contributed to the fact that Charrière was nominated to become officer of the Legion d'Honneur.

Another case of litigation has been described in great details - the subject of litigation was the incisor of the bladder neck. This time Leroy d'Etiolles waged a raucous conflict with Dr. Mercier.

In 1825 Leroy d'Etiolle published his book *Exposé des moyens de guérir de la pierre sans recourir à l'operation de la taille*, "Treatise on a stone removal without cutting the stone", which was followed by a number of publications at the Academy of Sciences on remedies to treat urine retention. His suggestions basically concerned the excision and scarification or the incision of obstacles developed at the bladder neck. The incisor or scarificator was constructed on the same principle as the lithomètre developed in 1825 which aimed at measuring the bladder stones. It also had the same basic construction as the lithotriptor with the difference that the male branch was not indented but had a cutting edge.

The first scarificator was manufactured by a mechanic called Greiling, the later models - by Mr. Charrière. In the years 1838-1839 Leroy d'Etiolles applied the incisor on his patients demonstrating the treatment to several physicians. Dr. Magendie from the Academy of Sciences confirmed this successful treatment with the incisor at one or two blades (Fig. 5).

In 1847, Leory'd'Etiolles modified the incisor by simplifying its structure to only one blade: He enabled the same blade to come out of both the convex and the concave side of the beque. He entrusted this idea to his instrument maker Mr. Charrière and to facilitate the manufacture he left a model with Mr. Charrière's craftsman, Mr. George Endler.

To Leroy d'Etiolle's surprise and anger two almost identically looking instruments - except for the handle one in metal the other in ebony - were fabricated in Mr. Charriere's workshop: one for himself and one for Dr. Mercier who claimed priority on this instrument. Not possessing any definitive proofs Leroy d'Etiolles strongly suspected Charrière to have transferred his ideas on the instrument to Mercier although Mercier maintained that the idea of this form of incisor had come spontaneously to him. Mr. Charrière's possible disloyal attitude also entailed some financial losses for Leroy d'Etiolles. It was not him, but rather Dr. Mercier who was proposed for the award by the Academy of Sciences. The so-called *Prix d'Argenteuil* was granted to Dr. Mercier for his research done on the treatment of urine retention by incision into the bladder neck.

Consequently Leory d'Etiolles deposited financial demands and also requested the restitution of certain instruments which were given to Mr. Charrière as models. The final court verdict on this litigation was not recorded in the minutes of proceedings[4].

The plaint raised by Leroy d'Etiolles accurately documents the two positions of the partners: on the one hand, there is the surgeon or physician as the representative of science - on the other hand, the instrument maker as the representative of business.

In analysing the conflict between Leroy d'Etiolles and Charrière one inevitably raises the following questions: was Leroy d'Etiolles's accusation of Charrière's disloyal attitude justified? Did he possess the exclusive right on Charrière's

4
Procès entre M. Leroy d'Etiolles, Docteur en Médecine et M. Charrière, Fabricant d'Instruments de Chirurgie. Bibliothèque Nationale, Paris, 1852.

products? What were the duties and rights of the instrument maker?

Such conflicting situations between physicians or surgeons and instrument makers have occurred more than once in the history of medicine. However, the cooperation between them has always been an indispensable prerequisite for technical progress.

Correspondence to:
Michaela Zykan
Internationale Nitze-Leiter Forschungsgesellschaft
für Endoskopie
Währinger Straße 25
A-1090 Vienna
E-mail: michaela.zykan@meduniwien.ac.at

CONTENTS of VOLUME 2
de Historia Urologiae Europaeae
(1995)

FOREWORD by F.M.J. Debruyne	7
INTRODUCTION by J.J. Mattelaer	9
THE HISTORY OF UROLOGY IN THE BRITISH ISLES by J. Blandy	11
THE HISTORY OF UROLOGY IN RUSSIA by L. Gorilovski	23
THE HISTORY OF UROLOGY IN AUSTRIA by H. Haschek	35
THE HISTORY OF UROLOGY IN ITALY by S. Musitelli, M. Pavone Macaluso, P. Marandola, M. Lamartina, H. Jallous, G.B. Ingargiola and A. Speroni	57
THE HISTORY OF UROLOGY IN BELGIUM by J.J. Mattelaer, W. Grégoir, A. Similon and J. De Leval	85
THE HISTORY OF UROLOGY IN POLAND by L.J. Mazurek	125
UROLOGICAL KNOWLEDGE IN RENAISSANCE SPAIN by R. Vela Navarrete	139
THE HISTORY OF UROLOGY IN SWEDEN by E. Lindstedt	159
THE HISTORY OF UROLOGY IN HUNGARY by P. Magasi	175

CONTENTS of VOLUME 3
de Historia Urologiae Europaeae
(1996)

FOREWORD by F.M.J. Debruyne	7
INTRODUCTION by J.J. Mattelaer	9
THE HISTORY OF UROLOGY IN FRANCE by A. Jardin	11
HIGHLIGHTS FROM THE HISTORY OF GREEK UROLOGY (from the late Bronze Age to the post-Byzantine period) by S.G. Marketos, A.A. Diamandopoulos, E. Poulakou-Rebelakou and C. Dimopoulos	35
THE HISTORY OF UROLOGY IN THE NETHERLANDS by J.D.M. De Vries	65
THE HISTORY OF UROLOGY IN CROATIA by D. Derezig	111
THE HISTORY OF UROLOGY IN FINLAND by K.J. Oravisto	119
THE HISTORY OF UROLOGY IN ROMANIA by E. Proca	127
AN INTRODUCTION TO METHODOLOGICAL PROBLEMS IN THE HISTORY OF UROLOGY by S. Musitelli, H. Jallous, C. Marandola and P. Marandola	137
OUTLINE OF A CRITICAL SURVEY OF UROLOGICAL HISTORIOGRAPHY by P. Marandola, S. Musitelli and H. Jallous	175
THE HISTORY OF BLADDER CATHETERISATION by J.J. Mattelaer	201

CONTENTS of VOLUME 4
de Historia Urologiae Europaeae
(1997)

FOREWORD by F.M.J. Debruyne   7

INTRODUCTION by J.J. Mattelaer   9

THE HISTORY OF UROLOGY IN THE EUROPEAN COUNTRIES

THE HISTORY OF BULGARIAN UROLOGY   15
by T. Patrashkov and C. Kumanov

THE HISTORY OF UROLOGY IN PORTUGAL   23
by F. Calais Da Silva and A. Pinto De Carvalho

THE DEVELOPMENT OF UROLOGY IN DENMARK   37
by V. Hvidt and L. Lauridsen

THE HISTORY OF UROLOGY IN NORWAY   51
by B. Otnes

THE HISTORY OF UROLOGY IN SERBIA AND MONTENEGRO   65
by J. Nikolic and D. Konjevic

THE HISTORY OF UROLOGY IN GREECE   87
(from the post-Byzantine period to our days)
by S.G. Marketos, E. Poulakou-Rebelakou, A. Rebelakos and C. Dimopoulos

THE HISTORY OF UROLOGY IN SWITZERLAND   101
by D. Hauri

THE HISTORY OF THE E.O.R.T.C.   119
by M. Pavone-Macaluso and P.H. Smith

HISTORICAL TALES OF UROLOGY

UROLITHIASIS IN NON-MEDICAL BYZANTINE TEXTS   155
by J. Lascaratos, E. Poulakou-Rebelakou and A. Rebelakos

THE EARLY (SURGICAL) HISTORY OF BLADDER CANCER   163
by F. I. Chinegwundo

RESTORATION OF THE PREPUCE A HISTORICAL REVIEW   175
by D. Schultheiss, M.C. Truss, C.G. Stief and U. Jonas

ERRATA: 189
CORRECTIONS TO VOLUMES I, II and III
by S. Musitelli

CONTENTS of VOLUME 5
de Historia Urologiae Europaeae
(1998)

FOREWORD by F.M.J. Debruyne	7
INTRODUCTION by J.J. Mattelaer	9
THE HISTORY OF UROLOGY IN THE EUROPEAN COUNTRIES	
THE MODERN HISTORY OF UROLOGY IN SPAIN SINCE THE RENAISSANCE by E. Maganto Pavon and R. Vela Navarrete	15
HIGHLIGHTS IN THE HISTORY OF UROLOGY IN GERMANY by P. Rathert, F. Moll and D. Schultheiss	45
THE HISTORY OF UROLOGY IN ALBANIA by F. Tartari	75
A BRIEF HISTORY OF UROLOGY IN SLOVAKIA by V. Zvara, J. Breza, M. Hor˜nák	97
THE HISTORY OF UROLOGY IN MALTA by P. Cassar	111
HISTORICAL TALES OF UROLOGY	
PHARMACOLOGICAL TREATMENT OF UROLOGICAL DISEASES IN THE ROMAN EMPIRE by S. Musitelli, H. Jallous, P. Marandola	131
THE HISTORY OF THE URODYNAMICS OF THE LOWER URINARY TRACT by J.J. Mattelaer	161
CIRCUMCISION: A SYMBOLIC ACT? A HISTORY AND ATTEMPTED INTERPRETATION by M. Libert	179
LITHOTOMY: ONE OF THE MOST MACABER CHAPTERS IN THE HISTORY OF UROLOGY by J. De Moerloose	209
TABLEAU DE L'OPERATION DE LA TAILLE BY MARIN MARAIS (1725) by S. Evers	235
UROLOGIC REFERENCES IN THE HOMERIC EPICS by E. Poulakou-Rebelakou, A.G. Rebelakos and S.G. Marketos	249
DE HISTORIA UROLOGIAE EUROPAEAE INDEX vol. 1-5 (1998) by Sergio Musitelli	

CONTENTS of VOLUME 6
de Historia Urologiae Europaeae
(1999)

FOREWORD by F.M.J. Debruyne 7

INTRODUCTION by J.J. Mattelaer 9

THE HISTORY OF UROLOGY IN THE EUROPEAN COUNTRIES

THE HISTORY OF UROSCOPY 19
(is in fact the history of medicine in Europe till the XVth century)
by J.J. Mattelaer

THE HISTORY OF UROLOGY IN GEORGIA 57
by L.G. Managadze, G.A. Gzirishvilli, T.I. Shioshvili, Z.M. Chanturaia

THE HISTORY OF UROLOGY IN TURKEY 69
by V. Solok, M. Çek

A BRIEF HISTORY OF UROLOGY IN LENINGRAD 89
by L.M. Gorilovski

THE DEVELOPMENT OF UROLOGY IN LITHUANIA 101
by K.K. Jocius, H. Ramonas, J. Mickevicius

THE HISTORY OF UROLITHIASIS AND ENDOSCOPY IN ALBANIA 121
by F. Tartari

HISTORICAL TALES OF UROLOGY

UROLOGY AND URINE IN BERNARDINO RAMAZZINI 133
by P. Marandola, S. Musitelli, H. Jallous

ANDROGEN THERAPY AND REJUVENATION IN THE EARLY 20TH CENTURY 141
by D. Schultheiss, J. Denil, U. Jonas

TRIBUTE TO ONE OF THE PIONEERS OF GREEK UROLOGICAL HISTORIOGRAPHY: 165
DR. SPYROS NAOUMIDIS (1907-1998)
by S.G. Marketos, E. Poulakou-Rebelakou, A. Rebelakos and C. Dimopoulos

LETTER TO THE EDITOR: 175
CONCERNING THE ARTICLE "RESTORATION OF
THE PREPUCE: A HISTORICAL REVIEW"
by F. Sorrentino, M. Sorrentino

CONTENTS of VOLUME 7
de Historia Urologiae Europaeae
(2000)

FOREWORD by F.M.J. Debruyne	7
INTRODUCTION by J.J. Mattelaer	9
THE HISTORY OF UROLOGY IN THE EUROPEAN COUNTRIES	
THE HISTORY OF UROLOGY IN THE UKRAINE by S.P. Pasechnikov	15
CURATIVE ATTEMPTS IN ILLNESSES OF THE URINARY ORGANS IN MEDIEVAL ICELAND by C. Kaiser	27
FIFTY YEARS OF INTERSCANDINAVIAN UROLOGICAL COLLABORATION: A RETROSPECTIVE VIEW by Å. Fritjofson	39
HISTORICAL TALES OF UROLOGY	
LITHOTOMY IN THE 18th AND 19th CENTURIES by P.P. Figdor	51
ENDOSCOPIC LITHOTRIPSY OF URINARY BLADDER CALCULI by M.A. Reuter	73
THE HISTORY OF TROCARS by G. Seydl	85
LITHOTRIPSY IN AMERICA: TRANSFER OF THE TECHNIQUE FROM EUROPE (1824-1840) by J.M. Edmonson	95
CHARLES V: AN INNOVATING UROLOGY PATIENT by R. Vela Navarrete	109
HIGHLIGHTS IN THE HISTORY OF THE OPERATING MICROSCOPE by J. Denil and D. Schultheiss	113
ROBERT PROUST - AN EMINENT DOCTOR IN THE SHADOW OF HIS FAMOUS BROTHER MARCEL by R. Speck	125

CONTENTS of VOLUME 8
de Historia Urologiae Europaeae
(2001)

FOREWORD by F.M.J. Debruyne — 7

INTRODUCTION by J.J. Mattelaer — 9

THE HISTORY OF UROLOGY IN THE EUROPEAN COUNTRIES

UROLOGY IN ESTONIA PAST AND PRESENT — 15
by Gennadi Timberg, Harry Tihane, Heiki Kask and
Eldor Mihkelsoo

THE HISTORY OF UROLOGY IN THE REPUBLIC — 31
OF MACEDONIA (FYROM)
by Stravidis Aleksander

EUROPE'S INFLUENCE ON AMERICAN UROLOGY — 39
IN THE 19th CENTURY
by Rainer M. Engel

HISTORICAL TALES OF UROLOGY

VIENNA: A TREASURY OF THE HISTORY OF MEDICINE AND UROLOGY — 61

by Johan J. Mattelaer

THE HISTORIC INTERACTION OF ANAESTHESIA — 73
AND UROLOGY
by Friedrich Moll, A. Karenberg and Peter Rathert

MALDESCENSUS TESTIS - THE HISTORY OF OPERATIVE TREATMENT — 95
by Knut Albrecht and Dirk Schultheiss

A REINVESTIGATION OF THE SIGNIFICANCE OF — 109
"BOMBOLZINI" IN THE HISTORY OF ENDOSCOPY
by Peter P. Figdor

THE HISTORY OF URINARY TRACT INFECTIONS — 119
by J. O. Elo

JOHN HUNTER: FOUNDER OF SCIENTIFIC UROLOGY AND PIONEER IN — 127
THE FIELD OF UROGENITAL SURGERY
by K. Skrepetis and N. Autoniou

OTTO KNEISE: A PIONEER OF MODERN — 137
UROLOGY
by Jürgen Konert

CONTENTS of VOLUME 9
de Historia Urologiae Europaeae
(2002)

FOREWORD by F.M.J. Debruyne   7

INTRODUCTION by J.J. Mattelaer   9

THE HISTORY OF UROLOGY IN THE EUROPEAN COUNTRIES

THE HISTORY OF UROLOGY IN BOHEMIA - PRAGUE   15
by L. Jarolím

THE HISTORY OF UROLOGY IN SLOVENIA   27
by Sedmak Boris and Trwinar Bojar

EUROPE'S INFLUENCE ON THE DEVELOPMENT OF SOUTH AMERICAN UROLOGY   33
by E. Maganto Pavon

MODERN UROLOGISTS: WHERE DO YOU COME FROM?   51
By P. Marandola, S. Musitelli and D.Vitetta.

HISTORICAL TALES OF UROLOGY FRANZ VON PAULA GRUITHUISEN (1774-1852)   73
- HIS CONTRIBUTION TO THE DEVELOPMENT OF LITHOTRIPSY
by T. Zajaczkowski, A.M. Zamann and P. Rathert

FRANCESCO PAJOLA (1742-1816) - A PIONEER OF LITHOTOMY   87
by P.P. Figdor

THE HISTORY OF RENAL ANATOMO-PHYSIOLOGY   101
by S. Musitelli and J.J. Mattelaer

LEON KRYNSKI - EMINENT UROLOGIST OF THE LATE XIXth CENTURY   131
- CREATOR OF SUBMUCOSAL TRANSPLANTATION OF THE URETERS INTO THE
SIGMOID COLON
by R. Sosnowski, T. Chwalinski, T. Demkow, A. Sródka

A 10th CENTURY MEDICAL DEONTOLOGIST, ISHAQ IBN ALI AL-RUHAWI,   147
AND HIS STATEMENT ON BEVERAGES
by S. Aksoy and A.Verit

OPERATIVE UROLOGY AND THE HIPPOCRATIC OATH   155
by P.F. Kalafatis, K.B. Zougdas, F.J. Dimitriadis and M.P. Kalafatis

COMMENT   163
by S. Musitelli

LETTER TO THE EDITORS   165

CONTENTS of VOLUME 10
de Historia Urologiae Europaeae
(2003)

FOREWORD by F.M.J. Debruyne   7

INTRODUCTION by J.J. Mattelaer   9

THE HISTORY OF UROLOGY IN THE EUROPEAN COUNTRIES

THE HISTORY OF UROLOGY IN THE REPUBLIC OF BELARUS   15
by A. Strotsky

UROLOGY IN THE MARIA HOSPITAL IN HELSINKI, FINLAND   25
by J. Elo and M. Ala-Opas

THE PEREGRINATIONS OF THE LICHTLEITER   35
by J.J. Mattelaer, M. Skopec, R. Engel and D. Schultheiss

WOMEN IN EUROPEAN UROLOGY   41
by M. Ruutu, J.J. Mattelaer and members of the EAU Historical Committee

HISTORICAL TALES OF UROLOGY

JULIUS BRUCK (1840-1902) - HIS CONTRIBUTION   59
TO THE DEVELOPMENT OF ENDOSCOPY
by T. Zajaczkowski, A.P. Zamann

UROLOGICAL TECHNIQUES OF SEREFEDDIN SABUNCUOGLU IN THE 15th CENTURY   83
OTTOMAN PERIOD
by A.Verit, S.Aksoy, H.Kafali and F.F.Verit

EVOLUTION OF VASOGRAPHY DURING 20th CENTURY   95
by K. Skrepetis, N. Antoniou

CASTRATION FROM MESOPOTAMIA TO THE XVIth CENTURY   111
by S. Musitelli and J.F. Felderhof

THE PROOF OF PATERNITY: THE HISTORY OF AN ANDROLOGICAL-FORENSIC   135
CHALLENGE
by K. Albrecht and D. Schultheiss

TABLE OF CONTENTS Volumes 1-9   147

CONTENTS of VOLUME 11
de Historia Urologiae Europaeae
(2004)

FOREWORD by F.M.J. Debruyne	7
INTRODUCTION by D. Schultheiss	9
THE HISTORY OF UROLOGY IN THE EUROPEAN COUNTRIES	
THE 50th ANNIVERSARY OF THE FINNISH UROLOGICAL ASSOCIATION by J. Elo and M. Ala-Opas	13
ETHICAL PRINCIPLES AND PRACTICE IN PEDIATRIC UROLOGICAL OPERATIONS IN THE OTTOMAN EMPIRE by S.N. Cenk Buyukunal and N. Sari	25
HISTORICAL TALES OF UROLOGY	
HERMAPHRODISM AND ITS SURGICAL TREATMENT FROM ARISTOTLE TO THE XV CENTURY by S. Musitelli	39
SEMINAL STAINS IN LEGAL MEDICINE: A HISTORICAL REVIEW OF THE FORENSICAL PROOF by K. Albrecht and D. Schultheiss	51
THE UROGENITAL APPARATUS IN JUAN VALVERDE AND ANDREAS VESALIUS by S. Musitelli	65
WILLIAM CHESELDEN, THE FATHER OF LITHOTOMY by S. Wheatstone, B. Challacombe, P. Dasgupta	81
SIR HENRY THOMPSON: ARTIST, SCIENTIST, MOTORIST, GOURMET, TRAVELLER, NOVELIST, CREMATIONIST AND SUB-SPECIALIST UROLOGIST by J.C. Goddard and D.E. Osborn	91
NIKOLAJ A. BOGORAZ: RUSSIAN PIONEER OF PHALLOPLASTY AND PENILE IMPLANT SURGERY by A. Gabouev, U. Jonas, D. Schultheiss	107
GEZA ILLYÉS, FOUNDER OF HUNGARIAN UROLOGY by I. Romics, Z. Fazakas, G. Nádas	121
ERRATA CORRIGE by S. Musitelli	133
TABLE OF CONTENTS Volumes 1-10	135
CORRECTIONS TO VOLUME IX	152

CONTENTS of VOLUME 12
de Historia Urologiae Europaeae
(2005)

FOREWORD by P. Teilliac — 9

INTRODUCTION by D. Schultheiss — 11

THE HISTORY OF UROLOGY IN THE EUROPEAN COUNTRIES

THE HISTORY OF UROLOGY IN LATVIA — 15
by I. Smiltens and E. Vjaters

THE DEVELOPMENT OF UROLOGY IN SZCZECIN: HOW POLITICAL CHANGES INFLUENCED MEDICINE — 23
by T. Zajaczkowski and E.M. Wojewski-Zajaczkowski

CZECHOSLOVAK-SWEDISH-FINNISH UROLOGICAL SYMPOSIA HELD BETWEEN 1969 AND 1988 — 53
by V. Zvara and J. Elo

ESTABLISHMENT AND DEVELOPMENT OF MODERN UROLOGY IN SYRIA: FRENCH INFLUENCE AND SYRIAN INITIATIVE — 61
by A. K. Chamssuddin

HISTORICAL TALES OF UROLOGY

A BRIEF SURVEY OF THE HISTORY OF SCIENTIFIC MUSEUMS FROM THE 15th TO THE 18th CENTURY — 73
by S. Musitelli and H. Jallous

PALEOANDROLOGICAL ITEMS OF THE EARLIEST RELIGIOUS ARCHITECTURE: 9-10th MILLENNIUM BC — 91
by A. Verit, C. Kurkcuoglu, F.F. Verit, H. Kafali and E. Yeni

THE FERTILITY GODDESS, CYBELE, AND ANDROLOGY — 101
by C. Asvestis, A. Siatelis, D. Anagnostou, P. Karouzakis, E. Coralles and A. Tselikas

CHOCOLATE AND IMPOTENCE: AN HISTORICAL VIEW FROM EARLY SPANISH DOCUMENTS AND BAROQUE LITERATURE — 113
by R. Vela Navarrete

MALE GENITAL PATHOLOGY IN LEGAL MEDICINE: A HISTORICAL REVIEW — 121
by K. Albrecht and D. Schultheiss

HISTORICAL REMARKS ON THE DIAGNOSIS AND TREATMENT OF HYDROCELES — 143
by F.H. Moll and P. Rathert

THE LITHOSCOPE 153
by H-D. Nöske and E.W. Hauck

GEORG KELLING: THE MAN WHO INTRODUCED MODERN LAPAROSCOPY 163
INTO MEDICINE
by M. Hatzinger and J.K. Badawi

TERENCE MILLIN: A UROLOGICAL PIONEER 171
by D.M. Bouchier-Hayes

CONTENTS of VOLUME 13
de Historia Urologiae Europaeae
(2006)

FOREWORD by P. Teilliac — 9

INTRODUCTION by D. Schultheiss — 11

IN MEMORIAM: PROF. DR. LUDWIK JERZY MAZUREK — 13
by J. Mattelaer

THE HISTORY OF UROLOGY IN THE EUROPEAN COUNTRIES

THE HISTORY OF UROLOGY IN BOSNIA AND HERZEGOVINA — 19
by D. Aganovic

HISTORICAL TALES OF UROLOGY

A MAGNIFICENT CIRCUMCISION CARNIVAL IN THE EARLY 18th CENTURY — 37
OTTOMAN PERIOD
by A. Verit, M. Cengiz, E. Yeni, D. Unal

KORO – THE PSYCHOLOGICAL DISAPPEARANCE OF THE PENIS — 57
by W. Jilek and J. Mattelaer

MASTURBATION AND MASS DELUSION: THE STORY OF SPERMATORRHOEA — 75
by D. Hodgson

THE LEGACY OF SPERMATORRHOEA A COMMENT ON THE ARTICLE BY D. HODGSON — 95
by F. Hodges

THE UROLOGICAL FATAL DISEASE OF THE BYZANTINE EMPEROR, — 101
JUSTIN II (565-578 AD)
by E. Poulakou-Rebelakou, C. Alamanis, E. Koutsiaris, A. Rempelakos

HENRY DE TOULOUSE-LAUTREC AND JEAN ALFRED FOURNIER: — 111
A RELATIONSHIP ON CANVAS
by L. Fariña

JOSEPH DIETL (1804-1878) HIS CONTRIBUTION TO THE ADVANCEMENT — 125
OF MEDICINE AND HIS CREDIT FOR UROLOGY
by T. Zajaczkowski

A HISTORY OF CRYOSURGERY — 145
by S. Ahmed

CONTENTS of VOLUME 14
de Historia Urologiae Europaeae
(2007)

FOREWORD by P. Teillac	7
INTRODUCTION by D. Schultheiss	9

THE HISTORY OF UROLOGY IN EUROPEAN COUNTRIES

THE HISTORY OF UROLOGY IN ICELAND by T. Gislason	13

HISTORICAL TALES OF UROLOGY

THE HISTORICAL JOURNEY OF THE PHALLUS FROM 10,000 BC by M. Kendirci, Ö. Acar, U. Boylu, A. Kadioglu, C. Miroglu	25
THE URINARY TRACT IN GERMAN TEXTBOOKS OF LEGAL MEDICINE: A HISTORICAL REVIEW OF 200 YEARS by K. Albrecht, D. Schultheiss	43
UROLOGY AT NECKER HOSPITAL 1966: A SCANDINAVIAN VIEW by J. Elo	65
MASTERS OF MICTURITION: THE FULLERS OF ANCIENT ROME by J. R. Hill	79
HANS CHRISTIAN JACOBAEUS: THE INVENTOR OF HUMAN LAPAROSCOPY AND THORACOSCOPY by M. Hatzinger, S.T. Kwon, M. Sohn	95
THE MOMENT OF ENLIGHTENMENT by R.C.M. Pelger	103
SIR PETER FREYER: A PIONEERING UROLOGIST by J. P. O'Donoghue	113
THE ORIGINS OF SCIENTIFIC TREATMENT FOR VENEREAL DISEASES IN ATHENS IN THE EARLY 20th CENTURY by E. Poulakou-Rebelakou, C. Tsiamis, C. Alamanis, A. Rempelakos	121
JOHANN ANTON VON MIKULICZ-RADECKI 1850-1905): PROMOTER (OF MODERN SURGERY AND CONTRIBUTION TO UROLOGY by T. Zajaczkowski	135
THE HISTORY OF AN 85 YEAR OLD EUROPEAN UROLOGICAL DEPARTMENT by I. Romics, R. Engel, T. Stevens, P. Nyirády	165

CONTENTS of VOLUME 15
de Historia Urologiae Europaeae
(2008)

FOREWORD by P-A. Abrahamsson   7

INTRODUCTION by D. Schultheiss   9

THE HISTORY OF UROLOGY IN EUROPEAN COUNTRIES BERLIN'S INTERNATIONAL REPUTATION   11
By Rainer Engel

PIONEERS IN UROLOGY   15
By various authors

HISTORICAL TALES OF UROLOGY INFORMED CONSENT IN BLADDER STONE
TREATMENT FROM THE OTTOMAN ARCHIVES   27
By S. Aydın, A. Verit

CASTRATION: THE EUNUCHS OF QING DYNASTY CHINA: A MEDICAL AND HISTORICAL REVIEW   37
By M. Bultitude, J. Chatterton

THE GREEK AND ROMAN PHALLIC INFLUENCE IN MEDIEVAL WESTERN EUROPE   49
By J. J. Mattelaer

A BRIEF SURVEY OF THE HISTORY OF PEYRONIE'S DISEASE   73
By S. Musitelli, M. Bossi, H. Jallous

WOLFGANG AMADEUS MOZART A UROLOGICAL PATHOGRAPHY   95
By M. Hatzinger, S.T. Kwon

GENITOURINARY MEDICINE & SURGERY IN NELSON'S NAVY   105
By J.C. Goddard

LUDWIG VON RYDYGIER: HIS CONTRIBUTION TO THE ADVANCEMENT OF SURGERY AND HIS CREDIT FOR UROLOGY   123
By T. Zajaczkowski

STUDIES ON THE KIDNEY AND THE RENAL CIRCULATION, BY JOSEP TRUETA I RASPALL   155
By L.A. Fariña

A MODERN POEM IN LATIN ON THE PROSTATE   165
By J. J. Mattelaer

TABLE OF CONTENTS Volumes 1-14   169

CONTENTS of VOLUME 16
de Historia Urologiae Europaeae
(2009)

FOREWORD by P.-A. Abrahamsson   7

INTRODUCTION by D. Schultheiss   11

THE HISTORY OF UROLOGY IN EUROPEAN COUNTRIES

LEOPOLD CASPER, THE UROLOGICAL HERITAGE   15
By F. Moll and P. Rathert

COMBAT UROLOGY IN WORLD WAR II URINARY PATHOLOGY AT THE RUSSIAN   27
FRONT (191-1943)
By J.M. Poyato et al.

THE TUBERCULOSIS HOSPITAL IN HOHENKRUG, STETTIN DEPARTMENT OF   43
GENITOURINARY TUBERCULOSIS IN SZCZECIN-ZDUNOWO
By T. Zajaczkowski

IN THE SLIPSTREAM OF DR. KOLFF   67
By H. Broers

RESEARCH ON THE HISTORY OF EUROPEAN UROLOGY PAST, PRESENT AND FUTURE   83
By J. Elo, J. Mattelaer and D. Schultheiss

HISTORICAL TALES OF UROLOGY

CATHERINE DE MEDICI: THE CURE OF HER "INFERTILITY" AND SUBSEQUENT   105
CONTROL OF 16th CENTURY FRANCE
By J. Gordetsky and R. Rabinowitz

THE MANAGEMENT OF URETHRAL STRICTURES   119
IN ANCIENT INDIA THE ERA OF SUÇRUTA
By R. Nair et al.

HRÚTR HERJÓLFSSON: A VIKING TOO LARGE FOR HIS WIFE URO-OATHOLOGICAL   131
WORKUP OF A 1000 YEAR OLD STORY
By S. Buntrock and W. Heizmann

THE ETYMOLOGY OF CASTRATION AND ITS ASSOCIATION WITH   143
THE SELF-CASTRATING BEAVER
By A. R. Rao

THE MANAGEMENT OF PATIENTS WITH A URETHRAL ANOMALY A   155
DESCRIPTION IN A TEXTBOOK OF SURGERY PUBLISHED IN THE 18th CENTURY
By E. Yesildag and S.N.C. Buyukunal

WHEN THE PHALLUSSES WERE STILL GROWING ON TREES   167
By J.J. Mattelaer

2010
ISBN/EAN: 978-90-815102-1-9
Printed by Drukkerij Gelderland
Arnhem, the Netherlands
© History Office EAU

For extra copies of this series:
History Office EAU
P.O. Box 30016
6803 AA Arnhem
The Netherlands

Frontispiece:
Top left: Illustration from Semseddin-i Itaki's *Pictured Anatomical Books*
Bottom left: Posterior view of prostate and seminal vesicles from *Tractatus* by R. De Graaf
Right: Genitourinary illustrations from *Epitome* by Andreas Vesalius

No part of this publication may be reproduced, stored in a retrieval system, or transmitted by any means, electronic, mechanical or photocopying without written permission from the copyright holder.